SURVIVING THE STORM

SURVIVING THE STORM

A WORKBOOK FOR TELLING YOUR CANCER STORY

Cheryl Krauter, MFT

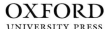

OXFORD
UNIVERSITY PRESS

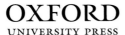

Oxford University Press is a department of the University of Oxford. It furthers
the University's objective of excellence in research, scholarship, and education
by publishing worldwide. Oxford is a registered trade mark of Oxford University
Press in the UK and certain other countries.

Published in the United States of America by Oxford University Press
198 Madison Avenue, New York, NY 10016, United States of America.

Library of Congress Cataloging-in-Publication Data
Names: Krauter, Cheryl, author.
Title: Surviving the storm : a workbook for telling your cancer story / Cheryl Krauter, MFT.
Description: Oxford ; New York : Oxford University Press, [2017]
Identifiers: LCCN 2016030166 | ISBN 9780190636166 (pbk.)
Subjects: LCSH: Cancer—Patients—Popular works. | Cancer—Patients—Rehabilitation—Handbooks, manuals, etc.
Classification: LCC RC263 .K68 2017 | DDC 616.99/4—dc23
LC record available at https://lccn.loc.gov/2016030166

This material is not intended to be, and should not be considered, a substitute for medical
or other professional advice. Treatment for the conditions described in this material is highly
dependent on the individual circumstances. And, while this material is designed to offer accurate
information with respect to the subject matter covered and to be current as of the time it was written,
research and knowledge about medical and health issues is constantly evolving and dose schedules
for medications are being revised continually, with new side effects recognized and accounted for regularly.
Readers must therefore always check the product information and clinical procedures with the most
up-to-date published product information and data sheets provided by the manufacturers and the most
recent codes of conduct and safety regulation. The publisher and the authors make no representations
or warranties to readers, express or implied, as to the accuracy or completeness of this material. Without limiting
the foregoing, the publisher and the authors make no representations or warranties as to the accuracy or efficacy
of the drug dosages mentioned in the material. The authors and the publisher do not accept, and expressly disclaim,
any responsibility for any liability, loss or risk that may be claimed or incurred as a consequence of the use and/or
application of any of the contents of this material.

9 8 7 6 5 4 3 2 1

Printed by Sheridan Books, Inc., United States of America

"When I left the hospital, I signed up for a call from a support group; that call never came. I live in a pretty isolated place and I remember feeling worried about my future and only the telephone connecting me with friends and family."
—Beth, cancer survivor

"It's a lot for a person to keep within themselves and it doesn't end when treatment is finished, it is an ongoing thing. It's a pressure, you want to comment about something to someone, a thought or a fear you may have, and the interest or response isn't there. So it would have been wonderful to have had somewhere to go and release some of these feelings. I believe there should be aftercare for cancer patients, one form being counseling."
—Suzanne, cancer survivor

"I think having a counselor with the ability to just listen would have been helpful."
—young cancer survivor posted on stupidcancer.org

"I have just heard that there are 450 patients on a waiting list at a major children's hospital for receiving outside emotional support."
—mother of a twenty-one-year-old cancer patient posted on stupidcancer.org

"We have three social workers who cover the entire population of the cancer center."
—Anonymous social worker at a major cancer center

In memory of my husband, John.
To my son, Ben.
And for all of you whose lives have been touched by cancer.

CONTENTS

FOREWORD: SURVIVING THE STORM

It's been almost a decade since that day in 2007 when Cheryl Krauter discovered a lump in her breast, and was referred to me, a breast cancer surgeon in Oakland, California. Cheryl was in her mid-fifties, a successful and busy psychotherapist, married, and the mother of a teenager. Simply put, she did not have time in her life for what followed—the biopsies, confirming the most aggressive form of breast cancer, so-called triple-negative breast cancer, already involving the lymph nodes under her arm; then surgery, chemotherapy, and radiation. But, like so many other women whose lives are forever changed by breast cancer, she made the time. Cheryl became a cancer survivor, joining more than 14 million other cancer survivors in the United States. A cancer patient becomes a survivor on the day of diagnosis and continues to be a survivor for the rest of her or his life. What separates Cheryl from other cancer survivors, is that after successfully defeating her cancer, she became determined to make life better for others dealing with cancer and its aftermath. Cheryl joined the ranks of the cancer survivorship movement.

Americans have a one in three chance of developing cancer in their lifetimes. Almost every one of us will have cancer or know someone close to us who has or had cancer. With improvements in cancer screening leading to earlier detection and with improvements in treatment leading to more frequent cures, the numbers of survivors increase daily. Many survivors, like Cheryl, recover with a renewed sense of life and purpose, but, unfortunately, and often unrecognized, is the toll taken by both the cancer and its treatment on health, functioning, sense of security, and well-being. Personal relationships change, and adaptations to routines and work may be needed. Importantly, the survivor's health—both physical and emotional health—is forever altered. Long-lasting effects of treatment may be apparent shortly after its completion or arise years later. Consequences of treatment can include the induction of new, and even different cancers, or chronic diseases that result from the toxic effects of the treatment. Cancer survivors often worry about whether or not the cancer will return, and, of course, it can. Complications of treatment can include chronic pain and alterations in anatomy and physiology, which can, in turn, result in inability to work and deterioration in relationships with family and friends. The social, psychological, and financial impacts of these changes can be devastating for cancer survivors.

In the months and years following her diagnosis and treatment, Cheryl experienced many of the complications of treatment that are commonly encountered. She had lymphedema (swelling and inflammation of the skin and soft tissues of the arm and breast associated with disruption of the lymphatic drainage pathways by surgery and radiation). She had chronic pain from neuropathy (inflammation of the nerve fibers resulting from surgery and chemotherapy). She had lumps develop in both breasts, as well as the changes of lymphedema, that were worrisome for recurrent or new breast cancer. She underwent fairly frequent diagnostic tests including imaging with MRIs and PET-CT scanners and blood tests and biopsies. She was tested for gene abnormalities that may be associated with breast and other cancers. Treatment for the lymphedema included compression, massage, medications, and acupuncture and for the chronic neuropathic pain, she received a variety of medications and acupuncture. Suspected infections were treated with antibiotics. Cheryl also had to deal with the psychological and sexual aspects of her disease, which she describes very clearly in *Surviving the Storm*, and their impact on her family, friends, and practice.

Cheryl describes her method of practice as "humanistic psychotherapy." Cheryl's focus is on the individual, her patient's problems, thoughts, fears, coping mechanisms, successes, and failures. I can't be sure exactly when or how she fully came to grips with her own cancer-related issues, but, clearly, she did. We then talked about helping others. I asked her if I could refer some of my own cancer patients to her for help. She was very graciously willing. The feedback that I got from my patients was always very positive, and I could see that they were clearly helped by Cheryl.

In 2011, I volunteered to develop a cancer survivorship program in Oakland and Berkeley, California. With financial and resource assistance from the Alta Bates Summit Medical Centers (ABSMC), we formed a working group of physicians (including surgeons, medical oncologists, radiation oncologists, gynecologists, family physicians, pain medicine specialists, and integrative care specialists), nurses, social workers, dietitians, physical therapists, hospital administrators, clergy, community organizers, and so forth—in short, everybody that I thought could help us deal with a multifaceted and growing issue in our community: the large numbers of cancer survivors, who, as the Institute of Medicine described, were being " . . . lost in transition."[1] There was only one person who I could think of with the experience, training, compassion, and skills to advise us on the psychological aspects of survivorship, and that was Cheryl Krauter. Cheryl accepted a position of leadership on our survivorship program steering committee and was instrumental in getting our program up and running, laying the framework to provide support and resources for our cancer patients and their families and friends. Our program's mission statement was very simple: to provide supportive services that optimize the health and quality of life of cancer patients in our community as they transition from treatment to recovery. Our vision was to achieve the mission by providing the essential components of survivorship care, including:

- A survivorship care plan (SCP) and treatment summary (TS)
- A health partnership that brings together the patient, primary care clinician (PCC), and the oncology clinical care team
- Access to resources that will promote a healthy and productive survivorship
- Continuous quality improvement of the survivorship program

We recruited people from our own community and from established circles of survivorship across the country to help us in our mission. These included Drs. Patricia Ganz and Kenneth Miller, pioneers in the survivorship movement, and the Journey Forward survivorship care plan software and development team, who made site visits, participated in symposia, and sat down with us, in person and in telephone conferences, providing us with their expertise and experience as we developed our program. Cheryl participated in these sessions, and her input into the psychological well-being of survivors was invaluable. Among our many achievements was the development of our own survivorship care plan that documented a patient's cancer; its treatment; and current ailments, concerns, and worries. We developed a specific plan for management of current concerns, follow-up guidelines, and, most importantly, assigned care providers to each identified task. We developed a distress level tool to serve as a baseline measure of the cancer patient's distress and subsequent progress. We conducted outreach to physicians in the community and educational conferences for the patients and the community's providers. We hired and trained full-time nurse practitioners to do the initial survivorship interviews and develop care plans and make and facilitate referrals to appropriate care providers. We developed, in partnership with UCSF Benioff Children's Hospital Oakland, a transition survivorship program for children who survived cancer and are now young adults.

When I retired from clinical practice, and as Medical Director of Survivorship, last year, the program was up and running and providing survivorship care plans to survivors in private physicians' offices and in the oncology clinics in the ABSMC campuses in Oakland and Berkeley.

There are still many challenges to be overcome in providing the essentials of survivorship care. Foremost among these is getting these services paid for. The Affordable Care Act (ACA) is a good start, but many people with cancer do not qualify for the services covered by ACA, and many of the services needed by survivors, including socioeconomic and psychological assistance are not covered. For the many cancer survivors for whom English is a second language, we desperately need to develop care plans with the help of providers who are fluent in the other common languages and cultures of our inner city community—we were working on these challenges at the time of my retirement, and I have no doubt that with the help of Cheryl and the other dedicated members of our survivorship community, they will be solved and the program will continue to evolve. Of course, our hope and prayer, and major research efforts, remain the elimination of cancer as a public health problem in America and the world.

Now, I invite all cancer survivors to read Cheryl's book and benefit from her experience and expertise as she helps you survive the storm.

Jon M. Greif, DO, FACS
Principal Investigator, Bay Area Tumor Institute,
a National Cancer Institute Community Oncology Research Program

NOTE

1. National Institute of Medicine, *From Cancer Patient to Cancer Survivor: Lost in Transition* (Washington, DC: Institute of Medicine and National Research Council, 2005).

ACKNOWLEDGMENTS

Before there was a book or even an idea of a book, there was my diagnosis of cancer. I want to thank my breast surgeon, Dr. Jon Greif, who is the embodiment of a humanistic provider. Not only did he guide me through cancer treatment, he was the first to give me the opportunity to form and present my ideas of quality survivorship care.

I want to express my gratitude to Linda Watanabe McFerrin, the mother of this project, for encouraging me to take what I believed to be an article and transform it into a book.

Thank you to Andrea Knobloch of Oxford University Press for championing the publication of *Surviving the Storm*.

With deep gratitude to Brooke Warner of Warner Coaching and She Writes Press, who has been my collaborative partner in the writing of this book. I'd like to dedicate a quote or a poem about her invaluable editorial support, but as it will probably only annoy her, I'll just say this: Not only did she help me make this the best book it could be, but along the way, she made me a better writer.

My appreciation to Meridithe Mendelsohn, PhD, for the supportive and inspiring conversations we began in 2009 and continue today, regarding the importance of quality survivorship care.

Thank you to Steve Ladd and Gabriel Ladd of Ladd Media for creating my websites and for helping me come online in the current century.

With appreciation to Patricia Eisemann, Vice President, Director of Publicity at Henry Holt and Company, for her generous guidance in the early days of this book.

I am grateful to be a part of the Women's Cancer Resource Center in Oakland, California, where I have been given the great privilege to work with a diverse population and become educated in the principals of cultural humility.

Thank you to my clients, students, trainees, and interns who have honored me with their trust and courageously shared their lives. I hope I have adequately expressed how much you have mattered to me.

I also want to acknowledge the people who generously agreed to contribute their stories to this book.

Some of my biggest fans and early readers are women who have believed in me and my capacity to write this book. Their love and encouragement kept me going. Loving thanks to Wilma Friesema, Bonnie Fluke, and Barbara Sapienza. A special thanks to Diana Wolf, who unfortunately died from cancer before she could see this book become a reality.

With gratitude to my mentor, James F. T. Bugental, PhD, who lives in every page of this book and is always with me as I sit with others.

Heartfelt thanks to my son, Ben, whose presence in my life makes all the difference. I owe a deep gratitude to my husband, John, who supported me through the process of writing this book, endured my lack of availability, listened to me rattle on about cancer, and, above all, always believed in me and what I had to offer. Sadly, he did not live to see the publication of this book.

SURVIVING THE STORM

INTRODUCTION

THE BLACK ANGEL BENDING OVER ME in the darkness of the cold, stark hospital room is the last to tend to me. Through an anesthesia haze I see the feathers of her wings lightly waving as she alights beside me. Her wingspan touches the bare walls enclosing me while I lie alone in the small metal bed. A breeze blows on my face; I look up and see kindness in her ebony eyes. Having lived with death in the corner of the room for years, this presence is no stranger to me. Has death come for me as this luminous raven woman, fluttering in disguise to trick me?

The angel's wing touches my arm and becomes a hand, gently stroking my arm. She whispers, "I have been through this; you will get through this, too." In that moment, she becomes the angel of mercy, the messenger of hope, the woman who has traveled the path before me and has reached her destination alive. Once again I have sent death skulking back into the corner to wait.

Not today.

The nurse, the woman, the cancer survivor finishing my care leaves feathers floating around me as I stare out of the drapeless window to an urban night sky with its wires, flashing signs, and empty buildings awaiting the occupants who will arrive at day's beginning. She will not return, but the touch of her winged fingers and her tale of resilience will remain, will be felt long into the years following this first encounter with the journey of cancer survivorship.

It only takes a few seconds to receive the news that you have been diagnosed with cancer—yet from that point on, your world has been changed forever. You enter a vast terrain of uncertainty, isolation, and insecurity when you finish treatment for cancer. What is it like to face daily life now that you are someone who has been diagnosed with cancer? Fear of recurrence, anxiety and depression related to uncertainty, loss and financial difficulties, and concerns around sexuality are all a part of this new territory. You may feel isolated, alone, and distressed. You have all the knowledge within you to understand and create your own healing, but sometimes you need guidance to help you find where you are and to support you in discovering where you want to go.

This book was designed to help you find your way through the wreckage of cancer so that when you land on new ground within yourself you will have ways to explore who you are as a survivor of the storm you have endured. No one handed me a map or installed a GPS when I left the treatment room. I just got in my car, drove to a bakery, purchased several pounds of pastries, and went home. I've talked to many people who have had similar experiences. This might sound familiar to you, too.

You have a unique story of your experience with cancer that can guide you and help make it possible for you to build an inner GPS that you can trust to show you where you need to be. I encourage you to draw your own map of the terrain you have inhabited to acknowledge the discovery of the ways you have been altered by your experience of cancer and document how you want to move on in your life. This deeply personal process of exploration is uniquely your own and does not bear the burden of proof of an evidence-based study; nor does it rely on any particular faith-based philosophy. This story belongs to you and in this book you are given a way to express the story of your experience with cancer.

> "Whether good or bad, life-changing situations often give people a chance to grow, learn, and appreciate what's important to them.
>
> Many people with cancer describe their experience as a journey. It's not necessarily a journey they would have chosen for themselves.
>
> But it sometimes presents the opportunity to look at things in a different way."
> —**National Cancer Institute,** *Facing Forward*[1]

In the spring of 2007, I discovered a lump in my breast. By the fall of 2007, I had undergone several surgeries and a grueling course of chemotherapy and radiation treatment. Even now those months feel unreal; I still wonder if somehow they had the wrong chart. But how could they make a mistake when they posed such questions as "What is your name? What is your birth date? Which breast is it?" I went from feeling fine to being in pain, horribly nauseated from chemo drugs, and burned by radiation. I watched my long curls fall into the tub drain. My mouth filled with sores. My eyes turned red. Too bad it wasn't Halloween; I was the perfect zombie. Scans, tests, blood draws, and MRIs became familiar, yet the feelings each one produced can still evoke anxiety years after the initial diagnosis. As I write this, I have no evidence of disease (NED).

As survivors, we are always waiting for the results.

I was fortunate to be able to continue my work as a depth psychotherapist in private practice throughout my treatment. I took time off for surgeries and was able to schedule my clients around the chemotherapy days when I was barely able to move and unable to eat. A kind radiation technologist agreed to treat me at a quarter to six each morning for five weeks so I could continue working. I am grateful to the clients, trainees, and students who were witness to my raw, bald vulnerability. I believe we all did remarkable and powerful work together during that time.

Part of the larger cancer trauma involves the serious cost ramifications. Some cancer patients are not able to work, and the economic implications of this can be devastating. Even though I was able to arrange a viable work schedule, I have not gone without making monthly medical payments since my cancer diagnosis in 2007, and I do not see any end to these bills. I know that I am not alone in this burdensome dilemma. And other patients may have difficulty arranging to take time off because of their job situations. I once read an article about a woman who was denied leave from her job because her breast cancer was not considered a life-threatening disease! The importance of addressing these common monetary concerns is essential throughout the difficulties of cancer, as they extend far into post-treatment for many people.

I believe that the treatment of the emotional trauma of cancer is as important as the treatment of the physical disease. Psychosocial support and psychotherapy are the pillars of healing for the survivors of treatment for life-threatening illness, as well as for the growing population of people who live with cancer. The capacity to look within and beyond cancer and the development of a strong self-advocacy are both key to healing and moving on with your life. When untreated, the emotional wounds of cancer continue to cause suffering that you do not need to endure. It is the medicine of the soul integrated with the medicine for the body that creates healing.

There is a great need for people who have been diagnosed with cancer to tell their stories—to share the real story of the emotional storm that is cancer, as well as the ravages of its treatments; to tell the tale of the cancer survivor who is moving from patient to person. You may not "feel like your old self," for it is not possible to remain who you were after the experience of facing life-threatening illness and the trauma of the treatment for that illness. The first year after the completion of treatment is a key time to explore and discover who you are after having faced the challenges of a cancer diagnosis. This is the time to begin the necessary process of self-awareness and self-advocacy to ensure quality for your survivorship care.

While it is confusing and frightening, your experience of finishing treatment for cancer can become a powerful opportunity to release trauma and move into a new stage of life. There are some survivors who continue with some form of treatment as they learn to live with the reality of managing cancer in their lives. The shadow of illness lingers. Some of the side effects of treatment are not visible and can be consequential—for example, ongoing pain from radiation, heart problems caused by chemotherapy, lymphedema, and scar tissue issues resulting from surgeries. "Chemo brain" is real and bothersome for people as they struggle with cognitive issues. I deal with sensory peripheral neuropathy, which was caused by chemotherapy and is not apparent until a shooting pain makes me wince or my balance goes berserk and I walk like I'm drunk. Though no longer always a death sentence, cancer can become a chronic illness. The growing population of survivors is misunderstood and underserved, particularly in regard to their emotional and psychological needs. There is value in addressing these needs and creating an avenue for care that is not merely a medical record but includes the heart and soul of cancer survivorship.

The term *survivor* is controversial and, indeed, there appear to be various definitions that are commonly used to describe someone who has been diagnosed with cancer. There's one that says you are a survivor the moment you have been diagnosed; another that says once you finish treatment, you are a survivor; there's the five-year mark, which seems to carry strong magical powers of defining a person's survival. According to the patients themselves, however, the sense of "I have survived cancer" may (or may not) come at different times in their lives.

> "I do not feel like a survivor. I can't seem to attach myself to that word. I am in remission. If I had been cured then maybe . . . but I am not."
> —**Pam T.**, cancer survivor

The threshold of the cancer experience that occurs at the infamous five-year mark of survivorship is another interesting place on the cancer recovery road. As I approached my own five-year mark in 2012, I experienced some pressure to "be over it." It came in subtle pushes to celebrate, as though I had accomplished something by still being alive. While I appreciated the well-meaning sentiments of congratulations and celebration, they left me feeling slightly empty and sad. I hadn't completed a project or won first place in a race. I hadn't accomplished something that I felt proud to cheer about. I didn't have a choice about having cancer—I'd had to react and respond. I was profoundly fortunate to have choices about treatment, to have insurance, and to have wonderful people who supported me. I am grateful for these past years since my diagnosis. But there's still no guarantee. I find this to be another significant juncture in cancer survivorship. It is a time for us to revisit where we are now and renew our intentions to fit this next phase of our lives.

This book marks the first phase of survivorship as the time when your treatment has finished, as well as the time period when an ongoing treatment regime begins. I have never met anyone who felt like a survivor at diagnosis or while undergoing initial treatment for cancer. Frankly, it's insultingly optimistic and reeks of denial. Surviving *with* cancer is a reality for some people. A recurrence of cancer can also throw a curveball in the direction of survivorship. The emotional impact that occurs at the end of treatment surprises us in unique ways; actually feeling like a survivor is personal to each of us.

While I am comfortable with the *title* of survivor, others bristle at the term, believing it to be too close to the former term that was commonly used: *victim*. Most of the other labels that are frequently chosen by those who have received a cancer diagnosis reference the experiences and terms of war, such as the "war on cancer." You don't usually see the "war on diabetes," or hear about a "heart attack survivor." Terms such as *warrior* and *veteran* seem to signify someone who has fought a hard battle and won. *Cancer conqueror* not only implies winning a hard battle but crushing the opponent and winning the war itself. Personally, my experience of cancer treatment was an assault both on my body and my psyche, and I believe the metaphors of combat speak to the ravages of cancer and its brutal treatments. The title of *reviver* might be the choice of someone who felt woken up by the experience of cancer and returns to the self profoundly changed. Younger and spryer cancer patients may call themselves *vixens*, suggesting a sexiness and a certain level of "in-your-face-cancer" defiance. As *survivor* is the most common identifier, however, I will use that term.

You may choose *survivor*, change it, or invent any name you want. Maybe you'll just choose to use your own name without any labels attached. What matters is that all of us who have weathered the experience of cancer feel that we have the space and the ways to express ourselves that feel real. There's a place for the vixens and the veterans!

I use the current definition of survivor to include the partners, families, and friends of the patient. At the center of the storm is the cancer patient—the person who has been diagnosed with cancer and is going through treatment or the person who is living with cancer. I am writing to and for you. But cancer affects all of you who are involved with the patient. You may not have cancer, but if you are in relationship with or caring for someone who has cancer, you are a person who's in the circle of distress and fear, which calls for healing. Attending to your needs as the partners, family members, and friends in regard to the trauma and emotional upheaval that you have experienced is as vital as bringing awareness to the needs of the patient. It is rare to find anyone whose life has not been touched by cancer, yet you can feel left out, helpless, and frightened, not knowing where or who to turn to. You need to tell your story, too.

I feel like I survived breast cancer, but I feel like I did not survive the treatment for cancer. I still deal with the long-term effects of chemotherapy and radiation. I know that this is common and, unfortunately, not always addressed in the years following treatment for cancer. This relates directly to quality of life for survivors. The following quote illustrates the impact of a cancer diagnosis and its treatment on the other survivors.

> "Mostly, I don't worry about her. I worry about my father, the rest of the family, should cancer return. I believe, without one doubt, that my mom could survive cancer again. I don't think my dad could."
> —**Jill, family survivor**

Quality of life is mentioned frequently in the context of cancer survivorship. While this is obviously subjective, it demands attention. There has been research indicating that the emotional recovery from cancer may not prolong life, but it will enhance *quality* of life.

This book uses the definition of quality of life from the University of Toronto Quality of Life Research Unit: Quality of life is "the degree to which a person enjoys the important possibilities of his or her life. Possibilities result from the opportunities and limitations each person has in [his or her] life and reflect the interaction of personal and environmental factors."[2] They identified three major life domains: being, belonging, and becoming.

The workbook sections in chapters 2 through 8 are included to help you reflect on your desired quality of life. The workbook exercises offer you, your family members, and friends an opportunity to tell your stories.

> "I would have appreciated having a survivor plan, which I understand is more common now."
> —**Suzanne, cancer survivor**

There are currently an estimated 12 million cancer survivors alive today in America. This population will expand as the baby boomer generation extends into the sixtieth and seventieth decades of their lives, making the need for comprehensive cancer survivor care even more significant. The type of attention needed for this group will differ drastically from the survivorship perspective of a pediatric cancer patient or that of patients in their late teens, twenties, or thirties. It is important to note that the estimated 12 million survivors only include those who were cancer patients and not the other survivors—partners, family members, and friends. These people have an experience in a different territory from that of the patient. Creating personalized care for the emotional needs of each of these different groups of cancer survivors gives a voice and a structure for self- advocacy and integrated care. Cancer is not a one-size-fits-all diagnosis, and neither is cancer survivorship.

You are not your diagnosis. You are not a statistic. You don't have to be a victim of a system that is overloaded and struggling to handle your needs. You can attend to your emotional healing as well as learn to advocate effectively for yourself in relationship to your medical team. You are at risk for numerous and varied physical, social, and psychological long-term effects from cancer treatment. Integrating your emotional needs into your life as a survivor is essential for your well-being. You did not create your cancer. It is not your fault that you got the short straw. You can find the light of transformation in the darkness of your fears and sorrows.

Imagine your story as a collage of pictures, pieces of hair and bone, a collection of tales from the road.

> No one discovers
> just where we've been, when we've been caught up again
> in our own sphere (where we must return, indeed, to evolve our destinies)
> —but we have changed, a little.
> **—Denise Levertov, "Sojourns in the Parallel World"**[3]

I wrote this book for the young woman in the oncology waiting room clutching papers of information about preserving fertility with shaking hands; she hadn't had that child she'd always wanted. This is for the woman who sat with me every morning at five thirty for five weeks at the radiology clinic, both of us there before dawn because we needed to remain at our jobs throughout our treatment for cancer. This is for the pale young man helping his father, who had just been given a death sentence, leave the oncology office to "get his affairs in order." This is for the woman whose story of cancer dates back twenty-five years to when there were no support resources for her to process the emotional trauma of her illness, and who still feels the aloneness and pain of that time in her life. It is for all the swimmers at the Oakland, California, Women's Cancer Resource Center's Swim a Mile for Women with Cancer, who plunge into the water each year to honor themselves and in memory of their loved ones. And it is for the young cancer survivors whose stories touch and inspire me.

This book is for the partners, families, friends, and colleagues who are sometimes not recognized as survivors. Your trauma can also find the voice of expression and healing.

This book is for the providers of services to cancer patients who work long and grueling hours and suffer from the emotional distress of constant contact with life-threatening illness.

This book is for my husband and my son, whose pale and terrified faces I looked up into after a surgery for breast cancer that didn't go as well as expected. It was in that moment that I knew that I couldn't give up, and I became a survivor.

This book is, with gratitude, for the winged nurse who was my first messenger of hope on the journey of survivorship.

This book is for the courageous clients who I am honored to sit with as they find their way through the storms of cancer.

As of yet, there is no cure for cancer . . .

NOTES

1. National Cancer Institute, *Facing Forward: Life after Cancer Treatment*, rev. ed. (Washington, DC: U.S. Department of Health and Human Services, National Institutes of Health [NIH] Publication No. 14-2424, 2014), 55.
2. "Quality of Life Model," Quality of Life Research Unit, University of Toronto, Ontario, accessed September 29, 2016, http://sites.utoronto.ca/qol/qol_model.htm.
3. Denise Levertov, "Sojourns in the Parallel World" in *Sands of the Well* (New York: New Directions, 1998), 49. Used by permission of New Directions Publishing Corporation. © 1994, 1995, 1996 by Denise Levertov.

SOMETIMES I THINK ABOUT IT

THE EXPERIENCE OF SURVIVORSHIP

1

She is being helped toward the open door
that leads to the examining rooms
by two young women I take to be her sisters.
Each bends to the weight of an arm
And steps with the straight, tough bearing
of courage. At what must seem to be
a great distance, a nurse holds the door,
smiling and calling encouragement.
How patient she is in the crisp white sails
of her clothes. The sick woman
peers from under her funny knit cap
to watch each foot swing scuffing forward
and take its turn under her weight.
There is no restlessness or impatience
or anger anywhere in sight. Grace
fills the clean mold of this moment
and all the shuffling magazines grow still.
—Ted Kooser, **"At the Cancer Clinic"**[1]

DR. M: "Five years from now you won't remember this."

ME: "Oh, I think I'll remember this five years from now."

DR. M: *(laughs nervously)* "Well, five years probably. But twenty years from now, you won't remember."

ME *(thinking)***:** Twenty years from now I'll be seventy-six years old . . . or will I?

FINISHING TREATMENT FOR CANCER IS LIKE falling off a mountain after your climbing rope has been cut. Well-meaning folks are cheering wildly, encouraging the celebration of such a monumental event. Some who have been there during the days, weeks, and months of the ordeal are frankly relieved that it is over and life can "return to normal." As you plummet toward what some call "returning to normal" or "the new normal," you realize that you are free-falling into some primal place of uncertainty, with no sense of where you are. You look up at the top of the cliff and see your doctors, nurses, and all of your caregivers waving kindly and a bit tiredly as they turn from you to face the next newly diagnosed patient. You're on your own; you hope you land in a safe spot. You might ask, "Hey where's my parachute?"

In his excellent essay "Restoring Emotional Well-Being," Robert Lent writes, "Surviving cancer does not just mean recovering one's physical health and adding theoretical years to one's life expectancy. It also entails coping with the many extra-physical (e.g., emotional, social, occupational, financial) issues that typically accompany—and may extend well beyond—that acute experience of cancer diagnosis and treatment."[2]

Five years after my diagnosis of breast cancer, I had not forgotten that I'd had cancer, gone through a grueling treatment, and was now in remission. I *did*—and still *do*—remember, as do others who have gone through cancer or continue to live with cancer. "Indeed," writes Lent, "in a recent survey of self-identified cancer survivors (most of whom had received a cancer diagnosis more than two years prior to the survey), 40% indicated that their life was still affected 'more than a little' by cancer, 53% replied that it was harder dealing with their emotional than their physical needs, 60% experienced problems in a close relationship, 32% reported job disruptions or loss, 72% reported suffering with depression at some point in their recovery, and 70% felt that their physician had been unable to help them with their nonmedical needs."[3]

It may be that it is important to remember our experience so that as we move forward in our lives, we have the opportunity to bring a sense of meaning and possibility with us. Life-changing experiences, while devastating and frightening, can become an integral part of our humanity, showing us a deeper part of ourselves. Sometimes we find places within us we didn't know existed, or we visit old familiar territory that needs to be explored in the service of more fully becoming who we are. Such are the openings and possibilities of surviving not only cancer but also the treatments for it, which may linger on for weeks, months, or years, and sometimes for the rest of your life. Your story matters.

"We are focusing on the number of people who are now alive who have experienced cancer at some time in the past, and their transition from treatment to recovery and the balance of their life," reports Elizabeth Ward, national vice president of intramural research at the American Cancer Society.[4] "But cancer survivors do have potential problems, including issues with quality of life and the need for both physical and psychological follow-up care. Cancer survival can affect one's life long term. Cancer survivors shouldn't feel abandoned after treatment has stopped."[5]

From the moment you are told that you have cancer, that the biopsy was positive, that those shadows in the MRI scan were malignant, and that the scan "lit up" with the colors of disease, your breath sucks in and stays there, landing in the pit of your stomach, where it will sit, unbelieving and stunned. You begin the journey here . . .

THE JOURNEY AHEAD OF YOU

The journey of post-treatment cancer brings challenges and opportunities. Minutes, days, months, and sometimes years after the completion of cancer treatment, feelings of loss involving the end of actively responding to the disease are common. Usually a significant amount of time and energy has been spent going to appointments and treatments, to the point that when the endeavor to obliterate those rogue cells ends, it can feel strange and empty. Having something to do in the face of life-threatening illness is oddly comforting, even in its horrendousness. The support team of doctors, nurses, technicians, family, and friends are present while you're in the eye of the storm and being held by that support team. As well as feeling a sense of power in fighting for your life, it creates a sense of purpose. There is a feeling of being watched; your surveillance team is on high alert. You feel an odd sense of safety. Then you are suddenly cut loose, still carrying the lingering physical and emotional effects of your diagnosis and treatment, and you embark on another phase of your life.

You may feel lost, alone, and unsure of the next step in the aftermath of cancer. "I remember feeling happy and scared," says Julie, a cancer survivor who was diagnosed as a young woman. "Happy that it was over, scared that my cancer would come back and no one would notice in time. My routine of regular blood tests [and so forth] seemed to fall off too fast. The information I got as to why they weren't needed as much seemed too vague. I mean, I had cancer, and now I'm supposed to walk out the door as if I'd had a routine infection or something?"[6]

While there are groups and workshops offered for survivorship, it can be difficult to navigate through a standardized mode of care. As previously mentioned, supportive services and learning-based workshops and groups are not uncommon; however, by the very nature of their structures, they are designed to provide a short-term, pragmatic approach. In all honesty, they are meant to be cost-effective and therefore desirable to a medical system that is running on a deficit.

Antiquated beliefs about psychological well-being still exist, creating a stigma about treating the emotional concerns of the cancer survivor. Assumptions and judgments form a bias that can be detected in scientific studies, as well as in the comments heard in the world of traditional, allopathic medicine. Those who express distress are sometimes identified as "anxious and depressed" patients. This diagnosis suggests that there is something pathologically wrong with those who experience distress when facing a life-threatening illness. Outworn and outdated, these value judgments only silence the distress and push it underground—the very place where anxiety and depression grow stronger. And this doesn't even begin to speak to those who face illness alone, without insurance, without many options, without much, if any, support.

In 1985, cancer survivor Dr. Fitzhugh Mullan wrote about his own experience with cancer in an article called "Seasons of Survival: Reflections of a Physician with Cancer," which was published in the *New England Journal of Medicine*.[7] In this piece, he identified what he called the "seasons" of cancer survivorship: "acute survivorship," which involves diagnosis and initial treatment; "extended survivorship," a time of watchful waiting with celebration, uncertainty, and transition; and "permanent survivorship," the season of gradual confidence that there will be a future free of cancer.[8] This groundbreaking work was the beginning of the recognition of the importance of the different stages of the cancer journey.

In December 2008, Kenneth Miller, PhD, co-wrote an article in the *Cancer Journal* entitled "Seasons of Survivorship Revisited." The writers said, "Many things have changed during the twenty years since Mullan described the 'seasons of survival.' Earlier diagnosis and better treatment have resulted in more people living through and beyond cancer, though more are able to live with cancer as a chronic disease. And although the intensity of treatment may result in an improved chance of survival, it can leave some survivors with late and long-term side effects."[9]

Miller and his coauthors go on to provide an updated version of the seasons of survival, identifying three categories. The first category is **transitional survivorship,** which is the time immediately after the end of treatment when patients are released from the treatment team. The second category is **extended survivorship**, which is the time after the transition from treatment (follow-up appointments, continued check-ups, tests, etc.), and includes those who are living with cancer as a chronic disease as well as those who are in remission because of ongoing treatment. The third category is **permanent survivorship**, which includes those who are in remission and asymptomatic and also those who are "cancer-free but not free of cancer" because of chronic late and long-term psychosocial problems. Miller and coauthors include in this last group those who develop second cancers as well as those who develop new cancers as a result of initial treatment.

The fantasy of permanency speaks to a level of control we all dream of attaining, attempting various methods and manipulations to figure out a way to achieve immortality. Impermanence is actually what we are all given to work with. I believe the term "impermanent survivorship" speaks to the concerns and thoughts of those who are faced with the shadow of cancer. Pam T., a triple-negative breast cancer survivor who has had recurrent cancer as well as serious side effects from aggressive treatment, speaks to this idea: "It would have helped if I had been able to turn to someone around me or had somewhere to go to talk about this horrible experience—also to learn of others' experiences," she says. "It is just a lot for a person to keep within themselves, and it doesn't end when treatment is finished—it is an ongoing thing."[10]

Having dealt with cancer and also having faced what it means to live a full life is both a gift and a curse. Allowing personal experience to be complex, both light *and* dark, transforms a dualistic, black-and-white way of thinking. By giving yourself the spaciousness to express—to yourself and then to others—what it is you need from your own experience of finishing treatment for cancer, you move more fluidly into the survivorship phase of your life.

WHAT HAPPENS NOW?

What happens now? What happens next? These are the questions that swirl in the mind and the heart of the survivor even before that last treatment. They begin to form without the knowledge of what is indeed next, or what will happen now. You are told about follow-up appointments, often given some advice on what to eat, and reminded to exercise. Most of this is common sense and applies to anyone attempting whatever the current definition of a "healthy lifestyle" is. However, while maintaining a healthy weight, exercising, and not drinking too much alcohol have been proven important, research remains inconclusive on the other effects of diet on cancer. Theories in the form of the latest product or program come and go, preying on us in our most frightened and desperate moments. Beware magic potions bearing promises of life everlasting!

Turning toward ourselves—reflecting on what to do now and what to do next, and exploring what is present—may fill the emptiness and soothe the terrors. It is not so much something to do, however, as it is a pathway to discover who you are now that you have survived cancer treatment. Deciding what's next may be as simple as deciding what you will have for breakfast, and it can also be as complex as exploring what you really want to do with whatever time is given to you. Asking the question, "What now?" may be an invitation to the awareness of who you are now as you stand at this crossroads of your life. Because there is little preparation for the emotional leg of survivorship, it can be confusing to know where to turn.

Leaning on others who can relate to your experience can be helpful during this time of transition. When asked what might have eased her anxiety immediately following the end of her treatment, Julie says that "a support group of survivors would have been good. I wasn't interested in continuing in a support group where people were still engaged in treatment. Done with that, sort of. But a group of people a number of years out, someone to say, 'Yes, I felt the same way. Yes, I bugged my doctors, too,' would have been good."[11]

Still tender from the shock of cancer, we stumble into the world outside the hospital and the doctor's office, shaken and unsure within ourselves and about our lives. "What happens now?" can be answered concretely by follow-up appointments, continued surveillance, medical tests, and so on. That's the short answer. But life has abruptly changed as the visits to the doctors taper off and another day arrives. The world has gone on without us while we were in surgery and in the infusion room and while we received radiation, and it will continue on with or without us. How we want to continue is a profoundly personal search. But it's difficult to begin to ponder these questions when it is still hard to believe that we *will* carry on at all. Working with these fears and beliefs may be the first part of "what happens now."

The answer to the first question, "What happens now?" can be separated into small sections, starting with day-to-day concerns and activities. For example, how do you want to use the time you have now that you've been freed from medical appointments and treatments? You may want to take a walk, read a book, nap, or paint. Start with what is accessible and easy; don't push or try to fit yourself into a place you don't really want to be in.

The answer to the second question, "What happens next?" springs from the first question. This involves introspection and reflection, not only about what has just occurred, but about what occurred prior to diagnosis and treatment. While there are many possible levels of inquiry, I am advocating a level of mindfulness that has depth. We will explore this in later chapters. The workbook sections in this book are written to evoke and encourage this type of self-inquiry and inner searching. Indeed, this book came from my own questioning of what happens next.

Just as there are different stages of survivorship, there are also different *ages* of survivorship. The needs of a child will not be those of a seventy-year-old person. The needs of young cancer survivors are distinctly separate from those of middle-aged individuals. Annette Stanton notes that "the most consistent demographic predictor of poor quality of life and unmet needs in adult survivors is a relatively young age. Depending on the developmental phase and cancer treatment regimen, specific challenges that are particularly acute for young cancer survivors include managing sexual and fertility concerns, depressive symptoms, concomitants of premature menopause, intimate relationships, and career goals."[12]

While all of us who have been diagnosed with cancer face challenges in post-treatment, there is a growing acknowledgment of the differences that you, as a young cancer survivor, face as you re-enter your life. In *It's Only Temporary*, Evan Handler's memoir about being diagnosed with leukemia at twenty-four years old, the author describes the unique experience of facing cancer at such a young age: "I felt cut off. Isolated. Friendships are generally based on shared experience.

I didn't know anyone my age who could identify with where I'd been, or even anyone twenty or thirty years older."[13] In addition to these feelings of isolation, pediatric and adolescent cancer survivors walk away from treatment with concerns of recurrence and long-term side effects that are vastly different from older survivors. Fertility issues are a stark reality in this group; you may not have a chance to make certain decisions about how you will eventually create a family. Many of you return to your peer groups with a sad maturity beyond your years. Your education may have been put on hold; you can feel like you are behind your friends and colleagues. Shame and distress over your appearance may occur just at the time when you are beginning to date. Partying when you can barely swallow water doesn't work all that well.

THE POWER OF TELLING YOUR STORY

In all the talks, workshops, and events that I have attended, as well as those at which I have been a presenter, I have found a great need for survivors to speak about their experiences—to tell their stories. As Pam T. explains, "Completing treatment doesn't close the door on that chapter of your life; you can't just dust off your hands and be done with it. The emotional and physical trauma remains."[14]

I have come to believe that the essential aspect of moving into survivorship in an integrated and holistic way is for all those involved to have the chance to tell their stories and to explore their inner world in a way that integrates emotional care into the other aspects of survivorship. There is a large amount of information that can periodically change and appear contradictory, making it difficult to plow through and understand. I watch eyes glaze over as another expert talks rather than listens. I have looked into the faces of fear and distress and have, myself, experienced similar things. However, my experience does not define yours, nor should there be a generic mode of treatment. While a standard treatment modality may be practical for emotional care, it just doesn't work very well. It is all too common for people to end up drifting back into an isolated state that does not promote healing and well-being.

A humanistic perspective expands beyond the learning-based, behavioral, and psychosocial resources that are currently available to cancer patients and their families and provides options that extend beyond the support group and medical models of treatment. A contemplative view opens up an alternative to the mode of tolerating or managing the issues of cancer and brings it into the realm of exploration, awareness, and acceptance. While it is tempting to find solutions and "fix the problem," there is much to be gained from moving toward the difficulties of the emotional residue of cancer. As Ondrea Levine writes in her book *The Healing I Took Birth For*, "It seems that one of my greatest teachers or teachings came from the times in my life when illness came upon me. The gift in the wound that illness seems to provide for so many is to remind the heart to move toward difficulties rather than turn away from them."[15]

We cannot expect personal treatment in an impersonal system. We cannot wait for someone else to advocate for us. Self-advocacy for cancer survivors is a process that can be learned by each one of us. It requires both information and introspection. Speaking up for yourself is the only way that you will have a chance of being heard.

If no one hears you, speak louder. As cancer survivors, we are millions strong, and if we all raise our voices, the noise we make will create one voice speaking up for our emotional recovery and healing.

> *Many things in the world have*
> *already happened. You can*
> *go back and tell about them.*
> *They are part of what we*
> *own as we speed along*
> *through the white sky.*
> *But many things in the world*
> *haven't yet happened. You help*
> *them by thinking and writing and acting.*
> *Where they begin, you greet them*
> *or stop them. You come along*
> *and sustain the new things.*
> *Once, in the white sky there was*
> *a beginning, and I happened to notice*
> *and almost glimpsed what to do.*
> *But now I have come far*
> *to here, and it is away back there.*
> *Some days, I think about it.*
> **—William Stafford,** "In the White Sky"[16]

NOTES

1. Ted Kooser, "At the Cancer Clinic," in *Delights & Shadows* (Port Townsend, WA: Copper Canyon Press, 2004), 7. Used by permission of The Permissions Company, Inc., on behalf of Copper Canyon Press, www.coppercanyonpress.org. © 2004 by Ted Kooser.
2. Robert W. Lent, "Restoring Emotional Well-Being: A Theoretical Model," in *Handbook of Cancer Survivorship*, ed. Michael Feuerstein (New York: Springer, 2007), 231.
3. Lent, "Restoring Emotional Well-Being," 231.
4. Steven Reinberg, "18 Million U.S. Cancer Survivors Expected by 2022: Report," *HealthDay*, June 14, 2012, http://news.health.com/2012/06/14/18-million-u-s-cancer-survivors-expected-by-2022-report.
5. Reinberg, "18 Million U.S. Cancer Survivors."
6. Personal interview with author.
7. Fitzhugh Mullan, "Seasons of Survival: Reflections of a Physician with Cancer," *New England Journal of Medicine* 313, no. 4 (July 25, 1985), 270–73. doi:10.1056/NEJM198507253130421.
8. Mullan, "Seasons of Survival," 270–73.
9. Kenneth Miller, Brian Merry, and Joan Miller, "Seasons of Survivorship Revisited," *Cancer Journal* 14, no. 6 (November/December, 2008), 369–74. doi:10.1097/PPO.0b013e31818edf60.
10. Personal interview with author.
11. Personal interview with author.
12. Annette L. Stanton, "What Happens Now? Psychosocial Care for Cancer Survivors after Medical Treatment Completion," *Journal of Clinical Oncology* 30, no. 11 (2012), 2. doi:10.1200/JCO.2011.39.7406. © 2012 by American Society of Clinical Oncology.
13. Evan Handler, *It's Only Temporary: The Good News and Bad News about Being Alive* (New York: Riverhead Books, 2008), 23. Used by permission of the author. © 2008 by Evan Handler.

14. Personal interview with author.
15. Ondrea Levine, *The Healing I Took Birth For: Practicing the Art of Compassion*, rev. ed. (Newburyport, MA: Weiser Books, 2015), 197–98. Used by permission from Red Wheel Weiser, LLC Newburyport, MA, www.redwheelweiser.com. © 2012, 2015 by Ondrea Levine and Stephanie Levine.
16. William Stafford, "In the White Sky," in *Stories That Could Be True: New and Collected Poems* (New York: Harper & Row, 1973), 217. Used by permission of The Permissions Company, Inc., on behalf of Kim Stafford. © 1973 by William Stafford.

A SECRET WORLD

THE INVISIBLE WOUNDS OF TRAUMA

2

Make no mistake. This will be an exercise in staying vertical.
Yes, there will be a view, later, a wide swath of open sky,
but in the meantime: tree and stone. If you're lucky, a hawk will
coast overhead, scanning the forest floor. If you're lucky,
a set of wildflowers will keep you cheerful. Mostly, though,
a steady sweat, your heart fluttering indelicately, a solid ache
perforating your calves. This is called work, what you will come to know,
eventually and simply, as movement, as all the evidence you need to make
your way. Forget where you were. That story is no longer true.
Level your gaze to the trail you're on, and even the dark won't stop you.
—Maya Stein, "How to Climb a Mountain"[1]

> "Each evaluation, breast exam, MRI, etc., brings me back to the terror of reliving the initial horror."
> **—Barbara, survivor**

A DIAGNOSIS OF CANCER IS A TRAUMATIC EVENT. While this is obvious at the moment of diagnosis and throughout the ensuing treatments, both the physical and emotional aftershocks that continue after the earthquake often go unnoticed and undiagnosed in the months and years that follow. Many survivors carry hidden scars, pains, neurological complications, and other invisible wounds for long periods of time—sometimes lasting for the rest of their lives.

The emotional scars of facing life-threatening illness can evoke a complex mix of fear, sorrow, anger, and confusion; the capacity to deal with the illness and all that it involves takes a massive amount of energy and courage. Yet even when you move beyond the illness, sensations, thoughts, and feelings still linger and emerge when you are vulnerable or tired, or when something triggers the invisible pieces of sharp glass or twisted metal still hiding beneath the surface of your skin, embedded in the soft tissue of your soul. This is what can happen when you have endured trauma, sometimes months and even years after the original incident. When trauma is denied, either by those who have experienced it or by others who cannot see or understand it, the wounds fester and grow, becoming like another cancer. It becomes a cancer of your inner world—a world where you struggle to breathe, feel that you can't move, and you're frozen in time. In the hidden depths of your secret world is a place that affects everything you do, everything you feel, and all that you are. Trauma can shatter your illusions of safety and control. When we can identify and then acknowledge that our trauma is congruent with our experience, we can move forward into a place of compassionate awareness. It's natural for you to feel traumatized. And it's helpful for you to explore and express your thoughts and feelings rather than to hold them inside, trying to "be strong and move on." It's okay to talk about what's happening with you and inside of you. When you name your wounds, you find healing.

Integrating the experience of trauma into your everyday life can be fraught with difficulties. What has happened to you is a part of you. It is your history, it tells about you. You are a person whose life story has a chapter titled "Cancer." And yet you don't want this chapter to be all that you're about. You want to turn the page. You want to write the next chapter.

How much do you share? What contracts within you and stifles your expression? Who are you protecting in your silence? How do you share your trauma with those who may be frightened by it? Your experience does not disappear, but how do you let the story become history and the wounds become scars?

Trauma is not objective. It is an inner, subjective experience that can only be truly known by the individual. Some people have gone through devastating horrors. It "makes sense" to define these as trauma and therefore they are easily acknowledged as such: diagnosable and acceptable, recognizable and treatable. However, when someone has an event that is not readily perceived by others as traumatic, they are often scorned, shamed, and invalidated. Simply stated, their experience is not believed by others. There is often a pressure to downplay the traumatic experience, which can lead to a kind of denial of your suffering. When this occurs, trauma may get buried; it may go underground and grow roots and tendrils of despair that sometimes take hold for an entire lifetime. Suffering in silence, the loneliness of living in a secret world is stark and raw.

The journey through treatment offers structure. It offers a road map and a set of directives, though this in itself is somewhat hideous because of the toxic nature of most cancer treatment regimes. After completion of treatment, physical trauma results from surgeries, harsh and toxic chemicals that have been poured into the body, and rays of radiation that have beamed into various tissues and affected bones and organs. The trauma to your body is often extensive and consequential, and side effects may linger for years. The trauma that lives in your body can be addressed, and this helps in the release and movement of the suffering you carry within. The emotional memory of your experience, however, lives in the dark realms outside your conscious awareness so that understanding the complexity of what you have undergone is subtler—more elusive to grab onto and understand. Yet by stepping into the light of awareness, you become conscious and find yourself on new ground. But what does moving on mean?

NORMALIZING THE TRAUMA OF CANCER

"People with histories of cancer are considered to be at risk for PTSD. The physical and mental shock of having a life-threatening disease, of receiving treatment for cancer, and living with repeated threats to one's body and life are traumatic experiences for many cancer patients."
—American Academy of Experts in Traumatic Stress[2]

The discussion of whether cancer and other life-threatening or chronic illnesses should be categorized as trauma is an ongoing debate in both the medical and psychological communities. The fifth and latest edition of the *Diagnostic and Statistical Manual of Mental Disorders* (*DSM-5*) excluded life-threatening illness as a category of posttraumatic stress disorder (PTSD).[3] Perhaps the acknowledgment of the stress and trauma of cancer is misunderstood in the traditional diagnosis of PTSD. The emotional complexity of facing life-threatening illness creates a controversial discussion of a standard PTSD diagnosis. Most of the research doesn't validate such a diagnosis and sometimes states that those who experience a high level of stress in dealing with cancer are those who are generally more anxious and depressed than the normal person. This is representative of the stigma that still exists concerning anything related to mental health issues, which can be mistakenly considered mental illness. Yet what a person endures through a cancer experience may not readily fit into a small box or a traditional diagnostic category. Your experience is more layered, personal, and therefore more difficult to categorize.

According to Cancer.net, there are "some aspects of the cancer experience that might trigger PTSD." These can include but are not limited to initial disease diagnosis or identification of advanced cancer; and pain, which can be caused by the cancer, medical tests and treatments, or any coexisting physical challenges. The test results themselves can cause the patient stress as can long-term treatments or stays in the hospital. And, of course, a recurrence of cancer can be very stressful for any patient.[4] Additionally, "people with cancer and cancer survivors who have PTSD need to have treatment because the disorder can keep them from getting needed tests, cancer treatments, or follow-up care."[5]

All of this information validates the trauma of a cancer diagnosis. While a clinical diagnosis of PTSD may not be warranted, the preceding statements clearly highlight the reality that from diagnosis through treatment and into survivorship, dealing with chronic pain, emotional distress, and possible disease recurrence makes it vital that stress and trauma be addressed. Moving beyond a cookie-cutter diagnosis and integrating humanistic approaches can more successfully attend to the traumatic experiences of cancer and its treatments and opens up the possibility for each individual's healing.

THE PERSONAL SUFFERING OF TRAUMA

> "The seven months of chemotherapy were the most difficult of my life. Chemotherapy was more than the treatment for my cancer; it changed me inside and out."
> —**Michele,** survivor

The damage our bodies undergo during treatment for cancer cannot be denied. The devastating effects of surgeries, chemotherapy, and radiology traumatize the human body. You know this, I know this. We have been there.

Secondary trauma caused by stress affects both patients and caregivers. Partners and family members of the patient experience high levels of stress related to what is occurring to their loved one, but often feel isolated and unable to voice their own trauma. Caregiver burnout is a significant issue that is only beginning to be addressed as a serious problem. Information pertaining not only to the side effects of treatment, but also to the possibility of late side effects and chronic difficulties, are too often not fully disclosed to either patients or to their support systems. I was told by an acupuncturist when I was in chemotherapy that it takes at least a full year to recover from the effects of that treatment, which was extremely helpful in my healing process. I now inform my clients of this and see the relief they experience after hearing this. Yet this information is not always clearly communicated by providers, leaving us in distress over lingering problems that can be misinterpreted and frightening. Some post-treatment medications have uncomfortable and consequential side effects including difficult and sometimes frightening mood shifts. Like a ripple from the initial trauma, these life-changing side effects affect both our emotional and physical well-being.

Don't feel crazy or strange if you experience flashbacks, nightmares, and repetitive and distressing intrusive images or other sensory impressions. It's common to experience strong feelings and reactions to reminders of cancer. My heart started racing when I got a call back for my mammogram and had to go in for more testing. In the twenty-four hours before I got the "all clear," my memories of the initial diagnostic mammogram were intensely vivid, as if the seven years that had passed were a mere seven minutes. Fearful monkeys ran rampant in my mind.

Not wanting to bring about scary or painful memories, you may want to avoid anyone and anything associated with your history of cancer, or those who remind you of unpleasant situations associated with illness. Conversely, you may find yourself obsessively checking for signs of disease and questioning anyone and anything incessantly. You might be hyperaware, or even hypervigilant, of perceived threats of illness. You may be irritable, have difficulty concentrating, or have trouble sleeping well. Or may you just feel detached and numb. These symptoms are normal; they are messengers from within connecting you to your thoughts and feelings.

> "For the first few years after treatment, not a day went by that I did not think about cancer and the cancer coming back. I had a heightened awareness of my body and became fixated on each minor problem. Each headache immediately prompted the thought, 'Is it brain cancer?'"
> —**Suzanne,** survivor

YOU'RE NOT CRAZY—OTHER PEOPLE FEEL THIS WAY TOO

It's important not to split your emotional trauma from the physical, as it creates a fractured experience that deprives you of real healing. Integrative care of distress addresses the whole person. When you approach trauma from a holistic perspective, there is no real separation of body and mind. By not breaking yourself into jagged pieces, you can heal more fully.

When someone listens deeply as you speak about what you are going through, where you have been, and where you are now, you are given the chance to let go and move on. Healing happens by being open to yourself as you are, not attempting to categorize, minimize, or dramatize. Trauma specialist Jeffrey Jay, PhD, writes, "in the books about PTSD the enormity of the victim's pain and horror is usually understated to make plausible the programs of recovery."[6] This relates to what can be a "dumbing down" of the dissemination of information to cancer patients. While this is understandable because of cultural fears of death and dying, as well as a misguided assumption that people are not intelligent enough to process on a more sophisticated level, it is condescending to the person who is facing life-threatening illness. Indeed, I believe it to be unethical to deprive human beings of the right to know, as best as possible, what may happen to them when they receive a medical diagnosis such as cancer. Informed choices are the right of each of us. After all, it is *your* odyssey.

Consider the healing of your trauma from cancer as a hero's journey. These sagas, by their very nature, are tales woven of dark and light threads. They speak of hazardous adventures where the good guy doesn't always win, love may not conquer all, and being good doesn't guarantee getting what you want. There are no shortcuts on this trail, but instead many loops, switchbacks, peaks, and valleys. The dangers that arise test the hopes of the hero who faces monumental roadblocks that question trust to its essential core. Most often the hero is reluctant and, given the option, wouldn't make the choice to take the trip, preferring instead to stay comfortably in the hut, or in front of the television. The call to adventure of your story happens with the diagnosis of cancer. It is at this moment that you find yourself on the precipice of a hazardous turn in the road. Looking forward, the choices you face, many of which lack clarity, will tangle together and crash into each other. In the confusion and fear of these early days, the unknown path before you is daunting. You may find yourself in a state of disbelief, thinking, "Surely they've got the wrong chart . . . who wants to travel this road?"

Most of us aren't rich and famous when we get cancer. While it would be amazing to step away into a beautiful restful place, many of us need to adjust our lives to this new reality of combating illness. We're just trying to get though each day, pay our rent or mortgage, and make sure the kids don't go off the rails. Ordinary lives plummet into extraordinary circumstances. I remember lying flat on the table in a dark radiology room, looking at the screen the radiologist had just turned so that I could see the mass in my breast, and saying, "Oh, I've got something to deal with." She replied, "Yes, I think you do." And life was never the same.

> "The most difficult aspect of [posttraumatic stress] PTS assessment in the cancer setting is the determination of precisely when to evaluate the patient. Diagnosis is complicated because cancer is not an acute or discrete event, but is an experience marked by repeated traumas and indeterminate length. Thus, an individual may exhibit the symptoms of PTS at any point from diagnosis through treatment, to treatment completion and, possibly, to recurrence."
> **—National Cancer Institute**[7]

FINDING WAYS TO HEAL TRAUMA

So often the end of treatment is marked as a celebration—"hooray, it's over, let's move on"—and then you might feel guilty because, in truth, you still really don't feel so good. According to Richard Tedeschi and Lawrence Calhoun, "some survivors report that they later view the trauma as an event that added value to their lives through forced changes, whereas others wish it could all be undone, given the sacrifices involved in achieving growth."[8] These varying thoughts and feelings once again show the deeply personal nature of the cancer experience. But what's true is that the event *did* happen, and that while the experience can become history, it will always exist. Perhaps those who "wish it could all be undone" might benefit from a further exploration of such a wish in order to better understand and maybe even in time accept their experience. It is possible that those who feel that the event added value to their lives are reporting the growth in survivorship that can come from hard lessons and the courage it takes to face them. In the end, feeling a sense of choice, power, and meaning helps you become enlivened regardless of the outer circumstances of your life.

> "Those who try to put their lives back together exactly as they were remain fractured and vulnerable. But those who accept the breakage and build themselves anew become more resilient and open to new ways of being."
> —**Stephen Joseph,** *What Doesn't Kill Us*[9]

It is important to allow time and space for the healing of trauma. All too often the push is for symptom reduction without attention to long-term concerns and effects. This is the post-treatment "management school"—how to *manage* stress, emotions, and grief. It's like getting a master of business of administration (MBA) in emotional management. But because emotions are not easily measured and emotional wounds are not as visible as physical wounds, managing symptoms without giving attention to underlying emotions will not take care of distress. This level of recovery can be misunderstood and rushed. Emotional recuperation is truly no different than recovering from a surgery or honoring the time it takes for the mending of a broken bone. Renewal is not necessarily quick, and real rejuvenation cannot be hurried.

The term *posttraumatic growth* has become another way to view and process trauma. What is posttraumatic growth? According to Tedeschi and Calhoun, "it's the experience of growth emerging from the struggle with major life difficulties [, which] can be successfully described by five major domains: seeing new possibilities, changed relationships, the paradoxical view of being both stronger yet more vulnerable, a greater appreciation for life, and changes in the individual's spiritual and existential domain."[10]

However, it is essential not to mistake this for a glib quick fix, a disguise using denial, or the avoidance that can happen with a "spiritual bypass." The psychological recuperation from any trauma is rarely without suffering as painful experiences are uncovered and relived. Like life, there are no guarantees that you will suddenly be without burdens, sorrows, and regrets. You can only choose how you will respond to what gets tossed at you. You may find a resilience within you that you never knew existed.

Bringing a raw honesty to the capacity for resilience when you are facing challenges opens a shattering clarity that lives within you, that *is* you. I have experienced a startling growth from having had cancer and have spoken with many others who have experienced profound life changes in survivorship. The mistake is to assume that the emotional challenges of the trauma experienced have a concrete beginning, middle, and end. Another misconception is that this will be fast and easy. You may be going along just fine and then something will smack you upside the head and a new layer of distress arrives—uninvited and unwanted. Again, the secret world may swallow you whole; you may say to yourself, "It's been years and I should be over this by now. What's wrong with me?" You have physical follow-ups for the rest of your life, why not emotional follow-ups as part of your survivorship?

> "It's just very stressful for people to be told that they have cancer. . . . You can't just assume that they feel bad now, but it will go away."
> —**Bonnie L. Green**, Georgetown University, Washington, D.C.[11]

As you negotiate the first weeks, months, and years of post-treatment, it can be traumatizing to schedule a visit with your oncologist, a laboratory test, a screening magnetic resonance imaging (MRI) scan, or a mammogram. Some days it's just difficult to keep going, let alone attempt a positive attitude. Some survivors find solace in their religious practices while others may have developed a spiritual practice that offers them a supportive perspective. However, not everyone is so inclined, and some people can have an isolative post-treatment experience when therapeutic or secular options are not presented and appropriate referrals are not made. It's not helpful to identify your distress if you are not given options that guide you in choosing how to effectively deal with your pain.

The distress *can* go away, but it doesn't just disappear. And distress may reappear. You didn't imagine your trauma, it's real. You don't have to be trapped within the darkness of a secret world. There is help. And it is okay to ask for it.

What helps? And where do you find resources and referrals? The resource section at the back of this book can help point you in the right direction.

Acupuncture, yoga, meditation, nutrition, massage, qigong, tai chi, and expressive arts therapies are offered by some cancer centers and clinics as a way to detoxify and heal from cancer. A great deal of suffering could be alleviated if these services were part of the treatment plan at the beginning of survivorship. Some hospitals and clinics have these services available on site. However, if this is not the case, you can ask your providers for referrals. Treatment for trauma, as well as psychotherapy sessions, are essential components of a survivorship plan that can honestly be deemed integrative. Holistic health must include mind, body, and soul in order to offer healing to the whole person.

> "In the attempt to improve our lives, we may urge ourselves with the familiar refrains: 'Just apply yourself . . . Start exercising tomorrow . . . Cut down on the sweets, booze, shopping . . . Pull yourself together . . . Come on, shape up, work out . . . You can do it if you really want.' And so it goes over and over again. These exhortations and good intentions are all admirable efforts at what we call self-control. While this ability is an important life skill, it is often modest in what it can accomplish and is fraught with obvious shortcomings. Frequently this strategy only works in the short run, leading us blindly into the quicksand of guilt and self-recrimination. Ironically, there are some days when it is no simple matter just to schedule a dental appointment or arrange for an annual medical exam."
> —**Peter Levine**, *In an Unspoken Voice*[12]

> "Anything that's human is mentionable and anything that is mentionable can be more manageable. When we talk about our feelings, they become less overwhelming, less upsetting, and less scary. The people we trust with that important talk help us know that we are not alone."
> —**Fred Rogers**[13]

WORKBOOK SECTION: IDENTIFYING AND WORKING WITH TRAUMA

How can you identify the trauma you may be carrying within you after a cancer diagnosis? There are signs and symptoms that help you recognize the moments when your thoughts and feelings are triggered. Your capacity to have an awareness of your experience can help you move from a triggered place of reaction to a more healing place of emotional response. Be sure that you are in a comfortable and safe environment as you review and respond to the following questions and exercises. If, at any time, the exercise feels overwhelming or too stressful, stop and take a break. Move at your own pace, paying attention to and honoring how you are feeling at each step. Remember that your thoughts and feelings are a natural response to the trauma that you have experienced.

I have included basic breathing tools to assist you in regulating your emotional reactions to trauma. This workbook section is designed to help you identify and self-regulate traumatic reactions. In that sense, it introduces you to the possibility of a deeper healing of the trauma you have experienced. I have purposely excluded more complex exercises or tools that are used to work with trauma as I believe it is important for you to do that work in a safe and contained space provided by an available and experienced clinician. Resources to help you find these providers are located in the resource section of this book.

How to Identify Traumatic Reactions

The following questions can help you to identify your reactions to any trauma you may have that's related to your diagnosis of cancer.

1. Do you sometimes have intrusive thoughts that are hard to let go?
   What sorts of things trigger these thoughts: smells, images, follow-up
   appointments, tests? What comes up for you and what's it like to deal with
   the reactions when this happens?

2. What helps you to be mindful of what triggers your traumatic responses?

3. Do you ever experience intense emotions or have moods that seem to dramatically change from moment to moment? Describe how this affects you.

4. Do you feel watchful or guarded in situations or with other people? This might mean that you are feeling hypervigilant, which is an extremely uncomfortable high level of fear. What's your experience?

5. Do you ever feel out of control of your body? This could show up as a racing heart or feeling cold, sweaty, or shaky. Comment on how this has happened for you.

6. Do you ever feel out of control in your mind? Do your thoughts fly off into the future, telling frightening stories of what might happen or create catastrophic scenarios in your head? How does this happen for you?

7. Have you ever experienced flashbacks of your cancer experience? What appears to you in these images?

8. Do you ever feel immobilized or numb? Feeling disconnected and shut down emotionally can be very distressing. Describe your experience.

9. What do believe about your capacity to move through and heal your
    traumatic experiences?

Listening to the Stories Your Body Tells You
BREATHING EXERCISES YOU CAN PRACTICE YOURSELF

Simple breathing exercises can help you to soothe and reconnect with yourself when traumatic thoughts, feelings, or images are triggering your emotions. You can practice working with your breath no matter where you are or what you are doing. These exercises are designed to help you regulate your reactions when you feel overwhelmed. You can do these breathing exercises with your eyes closed or open. The simple act of using your breath helps you to connect with yourself, and the more you practice, the easier it is to remember to check in with yourself in this way.

Exercise 1

Sit quietly.

Breathe through your nose.

Breathe into your center (your belly) and inhale all your energy.

Breathe out from your center and exhale all energies, distractions, anything that you don't want to carry.

Breathe in.

Breathe out.

Breathe in.

Breathe out.

Exercise 2

Sit in a comfortable position, or lie down in a comfortable place (whatever works best for you).

Place one of your hands on your stomach, just below your ribcage. Place your other hand over your chest.

Breathe in deeply through your nose letting the hand resting on your stomach be pushed out by your stomach. Notice that your chest doesn't move.

Breathe out through your lips, pursing them as if you were about to whistle. Gently guide the hand on your stomach inward, helping to press out the breath.

Slowly repeat three to ten times.

Exercise 3

This is a simple breathing exercise to help you sleep:

Lie down and make yourself comfortable.

Let yourself sink into the bed or floor and bring awareness to your body.

Feel how you are supported; relax any tension and soften with each exhale.

Focus on your breath and notice where you feel it in your body.

Take a deep, even breath into your center, hold for a couple of seconds, and exhale.

Continue this breathing pattern quietly and gently.

Allow yourself to soften and relax into your body.

Let your thoughts go with each exhale.

Continue your focus on your breath.

Let go.

Finding a Safe Place

It's possible to create a safe place within yourself that helps you to regulate your thoughts and feelings. You can develop a simple visualization or use your thoughts to build an affirmation that you can retrieve and use at any time. This is another basic tool to help you soothe yourself:

- Sit or lie down in a comfortable position. Close your eyes and remember a place where you felt safe and relaxed. Don't worry if you don't actually have an image; a memory or thought is fine. Let yourself be in this place. Slow down your breathing and become aware of how you feel in this place. You may want to bring another person or being into your safe place to comfort or guide you. It's up to you. Before you open your eyes, take a mental picture of your safe place so that you can return there any time that you want.

- Write down the story or draw a picture of your safe place.

Choosing Professional Guidance for Trauma Therapy

A common reaction to a cancer diagnosis is the feeling that your body has betrayed you. After your cancer treatment, you may be dealing with physical difficulties and limitations that are troublesome for you. Movement is considered helpful for the enhancement of both physical and emotional wellness and can improve relaxation and release traumatic reactions. You may choose to work with an experienced trauma specialist to help you regain your confidence and continue your healing process. Working with the release of trauma is evocative and it is wise to seek an experienced guide to insure that you are safe and well cared for as you explore these deeper issues. Always check with your healthcare providers and inform them of your intentions and the types of activities you are interested in.

NOTES

1. Maya Stein, "How to Climb a Mountain." Used by permission of the author. Maya Stein (www. mayastein.com) is a writer and creative arts facilitator currently living in northern New Jersey and graciously offered her poem for this book.
2. Amanda Chan, "One Third of Cancer Survivors Experience PTSD, Study Suggests," *Huffington Post*, October 15, 2011, updated December 15, 2011, www.huffingtonpost.com/entry/cancer-ptsd-symptoms-survivors_n_1008990.
3. American Psychiatric Association, *Diagnostic and Statistical Manual of Mental Disorders*, 5th ed. (Arlington, VA: American Psychiatric Association, 2013), 265, 271–80.
4. American Society of Clinical Oncology (ASCO), "Post-Traumatic Stress Disorder and Cancer," Cancer.net, January 2016, www.cancer.net/survivorship/life-after-cancer/ post-traumatic-stress-disorder-and-cancer.
5. ASCO, "Post-Traumatic Stress Disorder and Cancer."
6. Jeffrey Jay, "Terrible Knowledge," *Family Therapy Networker* (November/December 1991), 21.
7. PDQ Supportive and Palliative Care Editorial Board, "PDQ Cancer-Related Post-traumatic Stress" (Bethesda, MD: National Cancer Institute). Updated January 7, 2015, www.cancer.gov/ about-cancer/coping/survivorship/new-normal/ptsd-hp-pdq.
8. Richard G. Tedeschi and Lawrence G. Calhoun, "The Foundations of Posttraumatic Growth: New Considerations," *Psychological Inquiry* 15, no. 1 (2004), 93.
9. Stephen Joseph, *What Doesn't Kill Us: The New Psychology of Posttraumatic Growth* (New York: Basic Books, 2011), xiv, para. 2, lines 3–6. Used by permission of Basic Books, a member of Perseus Books Group. © 2011, 2012 by Stephen Joseph.
10. Tedeschi and Calhoun, "The Foundations of Posttraumatic Growth," 95.
11. Frederick Joelving, "Many Cancer Survivors Struggle with PTSD Symptoms," *Reuters Health News*, October 12, 2011, www.reuters.com/article/us-cancer-ptsd-idUSTRE79B7FT20111012.
12. Peter A. Levine, *In an Unspoken Voice: How the Body Releases Trauma and Restores Goodness* (Berkeley, CA: North Atlantic Books, 2010), 305–306. Used by permission of the author. © 2010 by Peter A. Levine.
13. Fred Rogers, *Life's Journeys According to Mr. Rogers: Things to Remember along the Way* (New York: Hyperion Books, 2005), 15. Used by permission of the Fred Rogers Company, 2100 Wharton Street, Suite 700, Pittsburg, PA.

LAYERS

THE PROCESS OF INNER SEARCHING

3

In my darkest night,
when the moon was covered
and I roamed through wreckage,
a nimbus-clouded voice
directed me:
"Live in the layers,
not on the litter."
Though I lack the art
to decipher it,
no doubt the next chapter
in my book of transformations
is already written.
I am not done with my changes.
—Stanley Kunitz, "The Layers"[1]

YOUR LAYERS ARE YOUR COMPLEXITIES, like rings that tell the age of the tree or paint that covers an original masterpiece. In the wreckage that is cancer, you can become trapped in the "litter" until you plunge deep beneath the surface to find what treasures and truths live within you. You uncover bits and pieces of artifacts you may never have dreamed existed within you; you discover the person you have forgotten, the one you aspire to become. You've drawn the short straw, but with it comes an opportunity to discover the heartbreaking clarity that appears when facing the *actual* possibility of your death. Waiting for you beneath the rubble may be a lucidity that cuts through old beliefs and habits.

In pulling off the layers of the familiar clothes that you put on to decorate and disguise yourself, you stand raw, much like being stripped bare in the operating rooms and the treatment centers when you are diagnosed with cancer. Those layers are cut, poisoned, and burned from you, leaving you to face the world in a new skin. You may be called to reflect upon the depth of your experience, to search within yourself to touch meaning and authenticity.

"Inner search therapies place more attention on what the client finds within the client's own stream of awareness when that stream is as little intruded upon (contaminated) as possible by the therapist. In inner search work, the ideal client condition is one of being intensely 'present'—that is, genuinely and nearly totally in the moment and what is going on. The truly present client is totally caught up in delving

> into subjectivity. This delving—and this is the important point which is often over-looked—is not a matter of 'thinking about' or 'figuring out' one's self. It is rather an openness to discovery within, which is more similar to meditation or to reading an intensely gripping novel than it is to doing arithmetic problems."
> —**James F. T. Bugental**, *Psychotherapy and Process*[2]

What if you could bring this way of being present with yourself—facing your life and the challenges that arise—into the realm of cancer, illness, disease? Acknowledging what is set before you as it is and exploring without judging or attempting to fix is a different mode of dealing with difficulty. In doing this, you give yourself the chance to find your way in your own time and in your own way.

MY INNER SEARCH AND WHERE IT LED ME

When I was first diagnosed with cancer, I was told by several medical providers that I was now a cancer survivor. Not only did this not make sense to me, it annoyed me. I didn't even know whether I would be okay, and no one really knows who will survive and who won't with any certainty at all. And when I went looking for resources to help me go through this frightening experience, I was disappointed to come up so empty-handed. Major cancer organizations did not return my calls, and I had such a negative experience with one local cancer center that I did not go back. All of this left me to set out on my own.

Because I have lived my professional life as an existential-humanistic psychotherapist, I am a person who wants to dive deep, which is partly what drove my inquiry into my own cancer diagnosis. The solutions and existing formats that had been prescribed for me to follow were frustrating. They simply didn't work for me, so I searched for another way. I felt angry when people tried to tell me that I would be alright, and even angrier when it felt like I had to take care of them in my response—so I agreed I would be alright. Eventually, I did find a depth psychotherapist with experience working with people with cancer who had the capacity to help me process my experience in a way that was satisfying and helped guide me toward growth.

However, bald and feeling naked to the world before me, I was not really ready to begin to sift through the wreckage that was my breast cancer until years later. Even now, eight years later and counting, I am still digging and discovering. My first plan of action, not unlike most people when first diagnosed, was to figure out how I could "talk my way out of this," continue on with my life, raise my son, and live to see grandchildren. My son was fourteen years old at the time, so this clearly meant I had some serious talking to do. It was not a time to reflect, but to act. When I was diagnosed, I did not feel changed, much less transformed. I did not respond well to the common punch line delivered to cancer patients that the disease is a gift. In fact, no one I've ever known who's been diagnosed with cancer jumps up and down with excitement at the gift they've been given. Instead I felt like I'd been socked in the gut. I couldn't breathe.

The *gift* of cancer often relates to the suggestion that there are opportunities afforded to the patient for transformation, for life changes that become more urgent and somehow more possible because of a cancer diagnosis. But I had no perception at the point of diagnosis how life would change. All I knew was that somehow

I would be forever changed, but I could not have known whether that would be for better or for worse or what those changes would look like. Was I a different person in the moments following diagnosis? Would I transform into someone else in the years following those first terrifying moments? In the chaos and confusion that follows the first shock wave, I was not even thinking about survivorship. I was thinking of survival. I got busy surviving. My guess is that at the beginning of your experience with cancer you may also feel this way.

> *Is Death miles away from this house,*
> *reaching for a widow in Cincinnati*
> *or breathing down the back of a lost hiker*
> *in British Columbia?*
> *Is he too busy making arrangements,*
> *tampering with air brakes,*
> *scattering cancer cells like seeds,*
> *loosening the wooden beams of roller coasters*
>
> *to bother with my hidden cottage*
> *that visitors find so hard to find?*
> *Or is he stepping from a black car*
> *parked at the dark end of the lane,*
> *shaking open the familiar cloak,*
> *its hood raised like the head of a crow,*
> *and removing the scythe from the trunk?*
> *Did you have any trouble with the directions?*
> *I will ask, as I start talking my way out of this.*
> **—Billy Collins,** "My Number"[3]

Transformed by the brutal chemical warfare being waged in my body, I continued to move through the world, to interact, to shop for groceries, sometimes forgetting my appearance until I saw my reflection in the sympathetic and sometimes horrified eyes of others. I was startled when I looked in the mirror into my own eyes. It could have been worse: I had a nice head that I covered with various scarves, baseball caps, and, sweetest of all, a number of beautiful little hats knitted with love by a dear friend. Pale, thin, and more than a bit shaky, I forced myself to venture out into the everyday world, which at times felt strange and illusory. I had no eyebrows, no shelter for my eyes. Eyelashes hurt when they fall out, like hard, hairy tears. My eyes, the mirror to my soul, had no curtains, and my soul stood open to the world. I felt raw and excruciatingly vulnerable.

Stripped of old illusions of hiding from others, I chose to stare back at myself. Looking into the eyes of my mortality, I examined my life. I searched for what I still believed and endured the many small deaths of what I had believed I could control or, at least, figure out. What I know today is that I had to let go of a lifelong (arrogant) notion that I was capable of figuring everything out. The family fable of long life because of my superior genetics (grandparents living into their hundreds and parents lasting well into their eighties) crashed into a new reality and fell off Mount Olympus when I got cancer at age fifty-five.

I did not take pictures of myself when I had cancer and no one else seemed inclined to snap a photo either. But then I was required to get clearance from my son's school district in order to accompany his class on a field trip. The county offices where I needed to take my forms and be fingerprinted so that I could be cleared to accompany teens to events were gray, dilapidated structures filled with people whose moods matched the bleak grayness of their surroundings. Baseball cap perched on my hard-boiled head, I wandered into an office with the final paperwork that would allow me to receive my badge. I looked like Mrs. Potato Head. The woman behind the desk immediately recognized what was in front of her. Her own family had been riddled with cancer, she knew the look.

"Should I keep my hat on for the photo?" I asked.

"No," she said, "you take that off, you *show* what it is you are carrying around within you."

Her words touched me; she did not turn away and I felt seen. She told me about the experiences she had with her family members who had cancer and I would later realize that she, too, was someone who needed to talk to someone—she had stories to tell. Yet what lived beneath my hairless skull, what was buried in the wreckage of my inner world, proved beyond what I had ever imagined. I really didn't know what I was "carrying around" within myself. I'm not sure that I could even begin the search while still struggling through the diagnosis and the treatment. It actually may be true for most of us that, like many crises, the time for reflection is not until the calamity has passed. It is in the aftermath of the storm that we sift through the remaining rubble. When hundred mile an hour winds are lifting the roof off the house, we just need to hunker down and find shelter. The varied and complex feelings of survivorship can appear deep in the layers, sometimes years after the initial diagnosis and treatment. For those who continue to live with cancer, the experience may be ongoing. How do you sit with all of this and still move on in your life?

I offer this brief synopsis of my personal experience to share with you some of what I went through and hopefully to provide you with encouragement and support for peeling off the layers of your experience. My wish is that you will allow yourself the time and space to search within yourself in ways that work for you so that your own transformation is authentic and that you are able to find a gold nugget in the trash heap of illness.

> "Someone once gave me a box of darkness. It took me years to understand that this, too, was a gift."
> —**Mary Oliver,** "The Uses of Sorrow"[4]

THE NEXT LAYER: INSIGHT, CLARITY, AND CHANGE

> "A transformation lies ahead. Just as there can be no 'middles' or 'endings' without 'beginnings,' there can't be an 'after' without its 'before.' And we can't often begin to know where it is we've been until we've traveled somewhere else and are able to look back."
> —**Evan Handler,** *It's Only Temporary*[5]

Cancer changes you, but whatever has been altered doesn't seem particularly clear the moment you receive that diagnosis. Authentic transformation shows itself over time, when you pay attention, give attention, and allow awareness to emerge. The essence of contemplative work is to be met where you are, not where you think you should be or where others think you should be. To meet yourself at the edges of your own known world requires letting go into the unknown territories of your inner world. You have to trust your capacity for growth and "hang in." You allow yourself to discover the untold story within you.

> "So many of the people whom I see have learned to treat themselves as objects—and, at that, objects to which they only have mild attachment. They hurry past their inner experiencing in an effort to report fully and accurately on these objects, and they regard my attention to the subjective as quaint, kindly, and impractical."
> — **James F. T. Bugental**, *The Search for Authenticity*[6]

Counseling that addresses adjustment or coping mechanisms is concerned with reducing stress and accepting, and sometimes resigning, oneself to situations and solutions. It is useful in that the focus of therapy is often on concrete tools or tips that offer relief and repair. While this can be helpful for relaxation or behavioral shifts, this initial level of therapy speaks to what can be done. It involves actions which, ideally, will result in change. Therapy that addresses these issues is about doing. In that way, it is more prescribed and concrete and helps people handle what might be called symptoms rather than treating the core or deeper level of healing. This is often the first layer of psychotherapeutic exploration, and in order to truly heal, we must go deeper.

Beneath this first layer of our busyness and incessant doing are tiers of being. There is a common misconception that "nothing is happening" when there are no tangible signs of change. We mistake the stillness required for reflection as stagnation. We interrupt the process of integration with impatience. We forget that listening to ourselves and to others is an important part of being connected. What does it mean to be present within yourself? How do you find what matters to you?

The *process* of searching for meaning, searching within yourself, is more alive and authentic than most of the answers you think you already know. It's not about the solution or the end result, it's about the question, or more importantly, the *questioning*. Inner nature, being in the here and now, is a practice that is always changing and growing. Like life, nothing stops; there's always more. It is the embracing of the process that defines searching. Searching is an active, inner practice of self-discovery. It is both a solitary as well as a guided experience. It asks for a sense of presence.

Bugental wrote, "Presence is 'being there' in the purest sense."[7] It's a quality of being in a situation where your intention is to be aware and to participate as fully as possible. The intention is to become conscious in body and mind. Aliveness comes from being in the present moment.

Softening into yourself allows an accessibility to your inner experience. Rather than hardening yourself against fear, you acknowledge yourself right where you are. You allow what is happening for you to matter, to have an effect. You take the risk to trust your own vulnerability as a path to your awareness. You give yourself permission to be open and engaged. You find courage and a willingness to explore.

EXPLORING YOUR DIAGNOSIS OF CANCER
AS LIFE CHANGING

Life puts before us essential questions:

- Who am I?
- What is the life I have created?
- What is the life I want to create now?
- What does it mean to me to be fully alive?
- How do I understand and interact with the world around me?

The existential crisis that occurs when you face a life-threatening diagnosis brings these questions into a sharp focus and hurtles past theories and assumptions into a startling place of reckoning. By allowing yourself to open to the true home within you, the place where you discover yourself as all that you are, you find a ground to spring from during the highs and lows of your day-to-day life now and as you move forward. This inner subjectivity serves as a guide and support through chaos and uncertainty and helps you to make authentic and meaningful choices. From here, you discover your personal narrative—your story.

Humanistic and existential psychotherapies are united by an emphasis on understanding human experience and a focus on the client rather than the symptoms. Humanistic therapy looks at the themes of *acceptance* and *growth*. The major themes of existential therapy are *responsibility* and *freedom*. The belief is that you have the capacity for self-awareness and choice and that this growing awareness comes from your process of searching through the many layers of your consciousness. Existential psychotherapy places a focus on finding meaning when confronting the issues we all face as we live our lives: anxiety over uncertainty, loneliness, despair, loss, and finally death. The emphasis is on how we choose. By deciding to focus on your creativity, authenticity, and free will, opening to your own inner potential, you may find avenues leading to transformation and meaning in the face of uncertainty and suffering. Rollo May wrote, "the purpose of psychotherapy is to set people free."[8]

When you choose to delve into this level of exploration and self-discovery, you open up to vast frontiers within yourself. Not that there is a particular destination or an ending point providing "the answers," but the very process offers a deep and satisfying inner engagement that is personally meaningful and informs your life choices. You become the author of your story regardless of the external circumstances of your life.

While in many ways, this manner of self-exploration cannot be concretely prescribed, there are certain aspects of inner searching that become clearer as you become familiar with your own process of exploration. You become more comfortable with long and sometimes challenging stretches of confusion and uncertainty. You learn a lot about yourself on the road to clarity. Letting go of old beliefs about who you are and what you want, while at times disturbing, can give you fresh perspectives that are enlivening. Time becomes almost irrelevant when you move off your well-rehearsed script into a mode of improvisation. You may actually experience this as a release (and a relief) from the time-constricted bounds of your day-to-day world. The vision of who you are and what is possible expands.

This layer of introspection inspires insight, which then informs choices. Choice leads to action and actions lead to authentic change. This is the work of the truly transformational path. You can alter the story of your life regardless of all the things that are beyond your control. You can creative a meaningful personal narrative.

THE IMPORTANCE OF PERSONAL NARRATIVE

"Why are we so attracted to stories? My lab has spent the last several years seeking to understand why stories can move us to tears, change our attitudes, opinions and behaviors, and even inspire us—and how stories change our brains, often for the better.... [As] social creatures who regularly affiliate with strangers, stories are an effective way to transmit important information and values from one individual or community to the next. Stories that are personal and emotionally compelling engage more of the brain, and thus are better remembered than simply stating a set of facts."
—**Paul J. Zak,** "**How Stories Change the Brain**"[9]

Being met and deeply listened to while you tell your story is healing in and of itself. Through the simple act of telling, of being witnessed while you paint the pictures of your experience, you find a certain relief, a freedom in releasing all that you have held and carried within yourself. One of my favorite childhood stories is Dr. Seuss's *Horton Hears a Who!* This is a tale of a loveable elephant who thinks he hears cries for help. Rather than ignore the pleas, he searches until he finds a dandelion puff, which turns out to be the entire city of Whoville. Horton picks up the flower and holds it carefully in his trunk, protecting it even as all the other jungle animals perceive Horton to be some sort of crackpot. Naturally this causes them to want to destroy him, along with the flower he is so steadfastly protecting. Finally, all the inhabitants of Whoville gather to organize a final scream for survival. With the aid of a megaphone, the smallest Who in Whoville cries, "We are here!" and at last, and in the nick of time, their distress call is heard. About to be boiled in oil, Horton is exonerated and the Whos are saved! The tag line of the story, a phrase that repeats continually throughout the tale, is "A person's a person, no matter how small."[10]

Because the medical world is so big and unwieldy, you as the patient can get lost in the shuffle of paper, backlogged appointments, and phone calls. It's not unusual to feel like a tiny Who, screaming to be heard. You feel like a number because, in truth, you have become part of the mass of numbers of cancer patients. It can feel like no one really cares about you and the narrative that is your story. We could all use Horton to listen and help us make our voices heard. We want to feel like someone cares.

In 1927, Francis Peabody wrote in the *Journal of the American Medical Association* that "the secret to caring for the patient is CARING for the patient."[11] This is no less true today, almost one hundred years later. Human emotions are universal and unchanging—only medical treatments change. We feel cared for when someone listens to us—when they listen to our story and have empathy for our experience.

A big part of my story was the choice to stay in the world of cancer by becoming an advocate for underserved women and their families, as well as expanding my psychotherapy practice to provide care to cancer patients, survivors, and their communities. I didn't make this choice lightly because I knew it meant that I would stay in the treatment rooms, face the politics, and be constantly reminded of the collateral damage of cancer. And, honestly, I still needed and wanted an authentic and contemplative way to discover and process my own experiences. I kept noticing that when given an opportunity, people wanted and needed to tell their stories. Some had never been given the space to relate what had happened for them. Time after time, going to conferences, workshops, and lectures, I noticed that no one was really listening to the concerns of the patients. The cries of the Whos were falling on deaf ears.

The universal need to care and be cared for transcends class and culture. And, in the end, no study or statistic will ever replace the human necessity for comfort and care. Perhaps the essence of self-care is the space you give to yourself for reflection and the intention to become wholly who you are. The human being you are wants and needs witnessing and confirmation that your story matters, that "you are here."

> "When our choices are to live, to be, when we give actuality to that which is potential within us, then we express our courage."
> — **James F. T. Bugental**[12]

THE GIFT OF AUTHENTIC TRANSFORMATION

> "If you could imagine the most incredible story ever, it would be less incredible than the story of being here. And the ironic thing is that story is not a story, it is true. It takes us so long to see where we are. It takes us even longer to see who we are. This is why the greatest gift you could ever dream is a gift you can only receive from one person. And that person is yourself. Therefore, the most subversive invitation you could ever accept is the invitation to awaken to who you are and where you have landed."
> —**John O'Donohue**[13]

If you are reading this book, you have landed in a place where you are sifting through the layers of your experience with cancer. Certainly part of this involves facing the truth of your mortality. Bernie Siegel said, "An awareness of one's mortality can lead you to wake up and live an authentic, meaningful life."[14] This is the true gift of transformation that is possible with a diagnosis of cancer. It isn't given to you; you give it to yourself. This is the hard work of metamorphosis. You accept the invitation to roam the wreckage and awaken to yourself. We want to be whole; we want to be who we are. A holistic approach to our own humanity—our innermost potential—moves away from a medical model of illness, from pathology to self-awareness, beyond behavior into self-expression and creativity. When we are screened for distress, instead of feeling trapped, we climb out of the small boxes we are asked to check. We fly off the cliffs of uncertainty and land in a new place we will come to know and understand.

> "Very often people object that they cannot possibly change their lives in a positive direction. They correctly point out that they are very ill, or that they have deep commitments with others depending on them, or they say that society will not permit it. I have never worked with anyone where positive change and growth, change that would make a crucial difference in the individual's life, was impossible."
> —**Lawrence LeShan,** *Cancer as a Turning Point*[15]

WORKBOOK SECTION: GUIDE TO REFLECTION, INNER SEARCHING, SELF-DISCOVERY

How to Begin

> "Life is not a problem to be solved but a mystery to be lived."
> — **Gabriel Honoré Marcel**[16]

Stop for a moment, sit quietly, and check in with yourself. Without needing to change or judge anything, take a moment to become aware of yourself right where you are now. Notice body sensations, feelings, and thoughts. You may refer to some of the breathing exercises in the preceding workbook section in Chapter 2 to help you come into the present moment within yourself. Allowing yourself to be still long enough to listen to your innermost thoughts and feelings may feel strange at first. It takes practice to shift your focus from the external world to your own inner world.

Use the following open-ended questions to help yourself discover and develop an inner searching process that leads to both awareness and insight. Remember that being quiet doesn't mean that you don't have thoughts and feelings. It means that you're pausing to bring an awareness to what is present for you in the moment. Don't be concerned if you feel confused or if your mind is very "noisy"—just stay with yourself. Remember that you are not looking for answers so much as allowing yourself to explore your questions.

Questions to Help You Reflect

1. How do you listen to yourself? What do you notice when you tune in to your inner experience?

2. Name some ways that help you come into a reflective state, for example, meditating, taking a walk in nature, or sitting alone in a quiet place.

3. What questions do you discover as you move into a more introspective state?

4.   What are your concerns about cancer?

5.   What is the life you have created?

6. What is the life you want to create now after cancer?

7. What does it mean to you to be fully alive? What are your challenges with being fully alive as a cancer survivor or as someone who is living with cancer?

8. How do you understand and interact with the world around you? Reflect on how your thoughts and feelings may have changed after your cancer diagnosis.

9. What's it like for you to think about accepting the reality of having had cancer? What is this like if you are living with cancer?

10. Ask yourself, "Who am I?" Don't think or plan too much, just watch your responses and the images that arise. Let yourself be surprised by what emerges. This ancient reflective question can be asked over and over, each time revealing something new.

11. Write a statement that affirms your own valuing of inner searching and personal presence. This can be a way for you to give yourself permission to take the time and the space to honor your own self-exploration.

NOTES

1. Stanley Kunitz, "The Layers," in *The Collected Poems* (New York: W. W. Norton, 2000), 217–18. Used by permission of W. W. Norton & Company, Inc. © 1978 by Stanley Kunitz.

2. James F. T. Bugental, *Psychotherapy and Process: The Fundamentals of an Existential-Humanistic Approach*, 3rd ed. (New York: McGraw-Hill, 1978), https://books.google.com/books/about/Psychotherapy_and_Process.html?id=8LUKAQAAMAAJ. Used by permission of Zeig, Tucker & Theisen, Inc., www.zeigtucker.com.

3. Billy Collins, "My Number," in *The Apple That Astonished Paris* (Fayetteville, AR: University of Arkansas Press, 1996), 54. Used by permission of The Permissions Company, Inc., on behalf of the University of Arkansas Press, www.uapress. © 1988, 1996 by Billy Collins.

4. Mary Oliver, "The Uses of Sorrow," in *Thirst* (Boston: Beacon Press, 2006), 52. Used by permission of the Charlotte Sheedy Literary Agency, Inc.

5. Evan Handler, *It's Only Temporary: The Good News and Bad News about Being Alive* (New York: Riverhead Books, 2008), xiii. Used by permission of the author. © 2008 by Evan Handler.

6. James F. T. Bugental, *The Search for Authenticity: An Existential-Analytical Approach to Psychotherapy* (Manchester, NH: Irvington, 1981), 383.

7. James F. T. Bugental, *The Art of the Psychotherapist: How to Develop the Skills That Take Psychotherapy Beyond Science* (New York: W. W. Norton, 1987), 27.

8. Rollo May, *Freedom and Destiny* (New York: W. W. Norton, 1981), 19.

9. Paul J. Zak, "How Stories Change the Brain," *Greater Good: The Science of a Meaningful Life*, December 17, 2013, http://greatergood.berkeley.edu/article/item/how_stories_change_brain.

10. Dr. Seuss, *Horton Hears a Who!* (New York: Random House, 1954), 6.

11. Francis W. Peabody, "The Care of the Patient," *The Journal of the American Medical Association* 88, no. 12 (March 19, 1927), 877–82. doi:10.1001/jama.1927.02680380001001.

12. Bugental, *The Search for Authenticity*, 26.

13. John O'Donohue, "The Question Holds the Lantern," accessed September 27, 2016, www.johnodonohue.com/words/question. Used by permission of the John O'Donohue Literary Estate. © 2016 by John O'Donohue. All rights reserved.

14. Bernie Siegel, *Love, Medicine & Miracles: Lessons Learned about Self-Healing from a Surgeon's Experience with Exceptional Patients* (New York: HarperPerennial, 1990), ix.

15. Lawrence LeShan, *Cancer as a Turning Point: A Handbook for People with Cancer, Their Families, and Health Professionals*, 2nd rev. ed. (New York: Plume, 1994), 53. See also Lawrence LeShan, *You Can Fight for Your Life: Emotional Factors in the Treatment of Cancer* (Guilford, CT: M. Evans, 1980).

16. This quotation is attributed to Gabriel Honoré Marcel (1889–1973), a French philosopher and existentialist, although variations are found, which are attributed to other influential philosophers, such as Joseph Campbell and Soren Kierkegaard.

WHAT IF?

THE FEAR OF RECURRENCE

4

Mine, I know, started at a distance
five hundred and twenty light years away and fell as stardust into my
*   sleeping mouth,*
yesterday, at birth, or that time when I was ten
lying on my back looking up at the cluster
called the Beehive or by its other name
in the constellation Cancer,
the Crab, able to move its nebulae projections
backward and forward, side to side,
in the tumor Hippocrates describes as carcinoma,
from karkinos, the analogue, in order to show
what being cancer looks like.
Star, therefore, to start,
like waking on the best day of your life
to feel this living and immortal thing inside you.
—Stanley Plumly, "Cancer"[1]

THERE IS A MAORI PROVERB THAT SAYS, "Turn your face to the sun and the shadows will fall behind you." Your fears of a recurrence of cancer bring you face to face with the reality of impermanence, staring at the bright glare of the sun as you stand in the darkness of the shadows that surround you. The fear of recurrence is the fear of death. This is why there is more to surviving cancer than surviving cancer. The door does not close behind you when you leave the treatment room. That door will be left ajar for the rest of your life. You are called to choose how you will walk through the numerous doors of your days for the rest of your life.

> "There is no cure (for cancer), so the anxiety of it coming back is an issue that is always on my mind."
> **—Pam T., cancer survivor**

These thoughts and feelings are common to those who have endured and moved beyond a cancer diagnosis and treatment. What has not been as common is the recognition of this distress as something that is unique to each of us and, therefore, responds well to a personal approach of care. These issues are of an emotional nature, and yet there is still some stigma around this being the territory of the unbalanced and that those individuals who are not prone to anxiety and depression prior to diagnosis will most likely move forward from their treatment without experiencing an ongoing distress, depression, anxiety and fear. First, this is simply untrue. Second, this allows little room for you to speak of your emotional distress and fears of recurrence. Something is *still* wrong with you. Not to pay attention to that truth is the "get over it" mode of healing. And that's okay for those who wish to step away from the experience and never look backward. But it doesn't cut it for the rest of us who choose to embark upon a personal search of healing and recovery.

Fear of recurrence lives in the mind and body of the cancer patient. Insidious secret cells of mass destruction hide in the silent crevices of bone and float in the stream of blood within. This is the shadow that follows every cancer survivor. The shadow spreads its dark cloud over both the patient and the others who stand in the circle around that person. This darkness is always present in the corner of the room, lingering a short distance behind you as you walk down the street or as you are brush your teeth before going to bed. It is your fear lingering, longing to be noticed, wanting to be told what to do, and looking to be comforted. How you choose to ignore or turn to face your fear depends upon the moment. *That you can choose* is the point. Both the capacity to look as well as the ability to turn away from this shadow allow for the potential to heal the emotional impact of treatment for cancer.

This fear, this sword of Damocles hovering over your head, is the essential concern that most of us struggle with after finishing treatment for cancer. These fears wreak havoc on quality of life as you transition from patient to person. There remains a lifelong struggle to reconcile these terrors as you travel beyond the initial phase of a cancer diagnosis. It is oftentimes difficult to find people who not only can support you, but actually help you to take the next steps into your life. Medical appointments become less frequent, others move on in their lives. Time in both its cruelty and kindness continues on without asking any of us for permission, or whether we're doing alright. There is a strong experience of vulnerability when you're in recovery, and if ignored, it prolongs your process of healing. This can be a confusing and lonely time. The fear of recurrence is a dark ghost wandering the many hallways of your mind.

In the night when your conscious mind is put to rest and the world of your unconscious comes alive, dreams may haunt you. The following dream is my own, shared here to illustrate the images that can arise when the conscious mind lets down its guard and the passageways of the unconscious open.

> I dream of rushing waters carrying bits of debris away from the river bank that I am standing on. A cold wind moves me toward the river, but I do not want to enter these swirling waters when I cannot see what is beyond the next bend. I look ahead to see lights trying to transform themselves into figures, and slowly the shadows begin to become my mother, my father, my grandfather, my grandmothers, my friend Richard. I now know that I am in the land of those who have died. In the distance, a brightness at once strange and familiar beckons and becomes Frank, a former partner who's passed on. I stand on the brink of the river of my ancestors and loved ones who have crossed over to the side of the river I cannot envision. I am on the edge of uncertainty. I am afraid and I weep and then lower myself into the river . . .
>
> I open my eyes. I wake up. My heart is pounding. I have made it back from the dark realms. I am still alive.

Fear of recurrence tosses those of us who are cancer survivors into a river of uncertainty. While every human being floats in uncertain waters, when you are moving on from facing a life-threatening illness, you have had an actual experience, a "brush with death" that is far different from a philosophical discussion of uncertainty and mortality. There is a stark difference between theory and experience, your thoughts and feelings are more real. The common feeling of being abandoned in a strange, unrecognizable land without a map relates to this experience of living with uncertainty. The rocky terrain of this foreign place is an uncharted territory waiting to be explored. It is a land that defies definition and explanation, a place to sit within a mystery that by its very nature you cannot fully know.

Anxiety and sometimes terror are experienced when facing the possibility of your own death. We like to think we are ready and not afraid to die, but these are largely stories we tell ourselves in order to cope with our fears. It is, perhaps, necessary to have these stories. They are tools to help calm and soothe ourselves. We can also spin tales of our disease recurring or being near death as a way to rescue ourselves from the anxiety of not having any control over what we fear might be secretly growing in our bodies. It can be easier to have the illusion that we have control of our destiny by directing all kinds of mental movies. Let's just admit that we all really want to control the show, and that we want the story to go the way we want. While it's both scary and frustrating to let go of the illusion of security, surrendering to the truth of uncertainty can be both the most difficult and most freeing thing we ever do.

> "Each person fears death in his or her own way. For some people, death anxiety is the background music of life, and any activity evokes the thought that a particular moment will never come again. Even an old movie feels poignant to those who cannot stop thinking that all the actors are now only dust. For other people, the anxiety is louder, unruly, tending to erupt at three in the morning, leaving them gasping at the specter of death. They are besieged by the thought that they, too, will soon be dead—as will everyone around them."
> —**Dr. Irvin D. Yalom,** *Staring at the Sun*[2]

COMMON QUESTIONS ABOUT CANCER RECURRENCE

In its publication "Living with Uncertainty: The Fear of Cancer Recurrence," the American Cancer Society defines cancer recurrence as "the return of cancer after treatment and after a lengthy period of time during which the cancer cannot be detected. (The length of time is not clearly defined.)"[3] They go on to list common what-if scenarios that survivors face:

- Will it come back?
- What are the chances it will come back?
- How will I know if it has come back?
- What will I do if it comes back?
- When will it come back?[4]

The common thread in all of these questions is the same: *What if it comes back?*

The fear of recurrence is all about whether we'll have to face again what we've already faced, what we'll do if that happens, and whether we'll survive the next round. Questions without concrete answers create fear for most of us. Yet these questions can become meaningful explorations of impermanence, too, which can grow into a new and powerful sense of what is possible in living with uncertainty. Moving beyond the management of feelings into the realm of deep exploration allows you to discover yourself in profound ways. Learning how to sit with the impossibility of predicting whether cancer will return speaks to the deep and disturbing fear of whether it will come back.

The "what ifs" are not only difficult, they're extremely confusing, because it's hard to separate out the aches and pains, the cough, or the back pain, from everyday ailments and something more serious. You might say to yourself, "Oh my God, I felt nothing the first time (I had cancer)." The chest aches and the heart pounds a bit faster in the early hours of the morning. Is the lump in the throat something I should call about? Has the pain in my lower back been there for more than two weeks? That's when they say to call. Instead a visit to the chiropractor relieves what is merely the usual disk problem. The skin rash is only eczema. You look fine and you feel okay. It's difficult because you don't want to seem like a hypochondriac, bugging the doctors and nurses, sensing their impatience with the small stuff. But then again, you don't want to ignore symptoms until it's too late. The questions of what to pay attention to, of when to make that call, and finally, when to insist upon that test even when the doctors (and the insurance company) don't feel that it is necessary, have no clear answers.

The medical advice to pay attention to our bodies is another balancing act of light and dark, attention and obsession. While clearly an important factor in being responsible, the focus on each pain, lump, and bump leads to confusion as well as anxiety and, for some, terror. There's a phenomenon in the cancer survivor community known as the "cancer pimple," whereby our fearful thoughts can create catastrophic stories about the possible recurrence of cancer upon the discovery of even the most innocuous of symptoms. Eating well and exercising are, without doubt, healthy for everyone, but to ascribe a magic property of immortality to them is a denial of the reality of cancer's willful and sneaky nature. For some cancer survivors, there is a loss of confidence in their body. A sense of anger, even outrage, that they have lived well, eaten right, and *still* got cancer.

One way to deal with "how you will know" is to, as best you can, know your own body. Be attuned to what you recognize as that old ache or the allergy that causes the cough. This speaks to working with body awareness so that when something unfamiliar pops up, you are aware of something that isn't usual. There are people who "had a feeling" that something was wrong, a dream, or intrusive thoughts or images. Someone I know had a dog who continued to scratch at her breast, the breast that turned out to be cancerous. Paying attention to these experiences leads to trusting your intuition, and therefore, developing that level of access to your health. Strong intuition is the key to the awareness of knowing your body.

> "The biggest change for me was the realization that my life might not work out as I had planned. My body had failed me, and I no longer had confidence that I was in control. I used to be confident about how my life would run. Getting cancer took away that confidence. Despite all I had done to be healthy, my body had failed me."
> —**Suzanne, cancer survivor**

> KYLE: "So what are your chances, what are your odds?"
> ADAM: "50/50."
> KYLE: "That's not that bad. That's better than I thought. If you were a casino game you'd have the best odds."
> —Will Reiser, *50/50*[5]

"What are the chances it will come back?" As cancer patients, we are given statistics in the form of a chart showing the percentage points indicating our survival statistics. First the chart shows us what are our odds are if we choose not to do whatever treatment is recommended. Then we get a second look at what our chances are if we do choose to enter treatment for cancer. Obviously this could be either an alarming or a hopeful process. Basically you get your grade in cancer (tumors are also graded, but in that case you really want a low, if not failing, grade.)

Statistics are not personal, they are not calculated to you individually, nor do they take into account whatever factors over which you have no control. Giving them too much power denies that which cannot always be explained or understood. Getting caught in the numbers game can derail the exploration of what your chances are and how you move forward. It's important to not put your life on hold. Watch that you don't stop yourself from taking risks or exploring what is meaningful to you. Regardless of the unknown quantity of the rest of your life, what is the quality you want for yourself in your life? The beauty of what is misunderstood as random may be the unexpected next step in your life.

And, let's face it. Numbers are a bit like trying to beat the dealer in Las Vegas. What are the odds? Hey, we're all on the bus to *that* casino!

The five-year survival rate refers to the percentage of patients who are alive at least five years after their cancer is diagnosed. Many of these people live much longer than five years after diagnosis, but the five-year rate is used as a standard way to discuss the prognosis (outlook for survival.)

> "There is another point to remember when talking about survival rates: Survival rates look at survival only, not whether the person is cancer-free 5 years after diagnosis. They are based on a group of people of all ages and health conditions diagnosed with a certain type of cancer. These statistics include people diagnosed early and those diagnosed late. As with any statistics, they should only be used to get an idea of the overall picture. They cannot be used to predict any one person's outcome."
> —American Cancer Society, *Living with Uncertainty*[6]

Statistics cannot be used to predict any person's outcome. "When will it come back?" becomes a question that leads to a process of releasing fear and ultimately letting go of control. Life, of course, does not come with a crystal ball, nor are we given any assurance of our "outcomes." For most of us, it is a struggle to let go, especially in the face of the fear of recurrence of cancer. Yet it is possible to move forward without the burden of constant worry. We are not sentenced to be prisoners of our own fear.

I have a strong memory of my first visit with my oncologist after finishing treatment. Still vulnerable and not at all convinced that this was over, that my cancer was gone, I asked him, "What will I do if comes back?" In his inimitable, irascible style, my doc said, "Then we'll go after it again." His matter-of-fact confidence combined with the honesty of not promising anything he couldn't deliver was strangely soothing. I believed him. Somehow those words sunk in and to this day, I believe that if I have a recurrence, I'll "go after it again."

FACING DOWN THE BOGEYMAN OF FEAR

You don't have to explore the "what ifs" alone. There are others with whom you can walk alongside, whether as guides or fellow travelers. Often these guides can be others who have had a similar experience with cancer themselves. Depth psychotherapists can also serve as guides down the raging river waters; they are psychological Sherpas through the high mountain passes who know how to navigate deep crevasses and avalanches. They do transformative work with the fear of recurrence—the fear of death—which does not involve fixing or managing experience. This kind of work instead explores the "what ifs" by opening the door to the root cellar and sliding down into the depths, providing a handrail and a lamp.

There are a number of ways to learn to be contemplative and to face yourself in an authentic manner. Often this involves simply slowing down long enough to listen to yourself, your thoughts and feelings, and the sensations in your body. Sitting with someone who can be with you and witness what you are experiencing without the need to change anything is helpful. By allowing your experience to unfold, you find your way through pain and trauma. Being with someone who doesn't need you to be different or to "get better fast" allows you to take the time you need to heal from within and to continue on with your life as it is now. As follow-up appointments and tests may extend for years beyond the original diagnosis, it makes it difficult to stuff your experience into a small box and close the lid.

Cancer centers and hospitals may offer groups, as well as individual counseling sessions, for those who have finished treatment. The support model is available for you if you choose to be helped in this way. This type of care can involve a short-term approach, which may include an educative program involving nutrition, exercise, meditation, and relaxation techniques. It is possible that a social worker will be present if you are in treatment at a hospital or large cancer center to help you with resources, referrals, and structure. Yet while navigation services may (or may not) be available while you are in treatment, it can be rare to find that kind of help after you have completed your treatment.

There is also a growing reliance on online support systems to provide help as well as a sense of community. Some relate to particular cancers while others are more general. I spent some lovely and touching time with the women on the Triple Negative Breast Cancer Foundation forum (https://tnbcfoundation.org/). I discovered them quite by accident and not only found support and reassurance but humor and friendship with others who were members of this group. I am on several Facebook groups that relate specifically to triple-negative breast cancer and find the contact engaging. There are times when we lose a member to a recurrence of cancer, and those are always tough, tender, and frightening moments. Indeed, when another person, whether it's a deeply personal connection or just an acquaintance, suffers a recurrence, there is a ripple in the surrounding waters.

I remember the last time I talked with my longtime dear friend, Diana. The recurrence of her cancer was like a bomb exploding in her body. It came fast and furious. Within a week she was slipping in and out of consciousness. Within five days she was unable to speak anymore. At the time, I lived more than eight hundred miles away and called to speak with her hospice nurse, who turned out to be a beautiful soul who understood my pain and grief at no longer being able to talk with a friend who had been in my life for thirty-seven years. The nurse brought the phone to Diana's bedside so that I could speak to her. As I did, she began to open her eyes. The nurse relayed what she saw to me as I continued to speak. At one point I began to laugh, saying to Diana, "Well, this is a first, me getting the last word in. That's never happened in our relationship."

The nurse, also laughing, then gasped and told me, "You won't believe this, but she is actually attempting to speak."

It was our last moment together. She died less than forty-eight hours later. Her death from cancer deeply grieves me to this day, and at the time, it brought up deep fears about recurrence. She seemed fine one moment, and then the next moment the cancer had won. The cancer had come back and taken her like a rogue wave. Not only do I grieve the loss of a dear friend but the way in which she was fine one moment and then within days, died, frightens me. It reminded me that cancer itself is a rogue disease that can rise up unexpectedly and carry me off to sea. I believe that most of us carry these fears within us.

> "The appointment upon completion of chemo, my oncologist was telling me if I have aches, pains, anything unusual that lasted for more than two weeks, to give him a call. My response was, 'OMG that is comforting . . . I felt nothing the first time (I had cancer) . . . by the time I feel something it'll be too late!' "
> —**Kirby,** cancer survivor
>
> "If I notice that I am breathing a little differently (due to the nature of having it in my lungs), I find myself wondering about that small possibility that my lymphoma could be making a comeback."
> —**Michele,** cancer survivor

How do we move through these fears so that we aren't paralyzed by anxiety? It's possible to transform these dark moments into rays of light. The sense of urgency that many cancer survivors feel is like a strong wave moving them forward. Things that have seemed vital and important are questioned; some are left behind on an old shore that has no use anymore. Sometimes this urgency is mistaken for the anxiety of death and wasted in moments of management that imply a "settle down" quality. An open heart and eyes turned inward pull the roots up, find the seeds, and plant them into the ground of growth.

A renewed passion for living life is possible. Some of us not only find ourselves trying something new, which is something we have always wanted to try, but also returning to interests or activities we may have left in the past. When faced with the "what ifs," we may choose to let go of ways in which we have held ourselves back, say, "What the hell?" and choose to take new risks and explore different paths.

> "I sat with myself and asked, if I had a year to live would I have regret? The answer was yes. I created something out of that exploration so that if I died right now I won't have regret. People who don't allow the impact miss something."
>
> **—Margie, cancer survivor**

> "Cancer still scares me. Each evaluation, breast exam, MRI, [and so forth] brings me to the terror of reliving that initial horror. My work continues to stay in the present moment, to allow my feelings, and to remember I am one of the women warriors who walk around with a heartfelt sense of what it means to be alive and to live fully in each moment. I have a strong desire to serve others and to make the world a better place."
>
> **—Barbara, cancer survivor**

The seeds of these women's experiences sprouted and grew beautiful plants after cancer. Both of them found that service to others gave their lives renewed purpose. Focusing on others is one avenue to address the transformation of fear.

But there are no real shortcuts to facing our fears. There can be both external and internal pressure to pretend that there is no fear or that there is some specified time in which you should no longer feel fear. This is not only unrealistic, it stifles the actual processing of fear so that there can be an experience of moving on that is authentic. Facing fears of recurrence and death, and breathing each breath through the walls of terror is not a light venture. Yet when you move beyond being a tentative acquaintance of fear and into a familiar friendship with those feelings and thoughts, you may discover a calm acceptance within yourself.

Giving power to fear—letting fear control you—controls your life and the choices you make. Fear is just another feeling in the multitude of feelings contained in your emotional palette. Accepting fear as merely another emotion in this palette of your inner world allows that experience to ebb and flow naturally. Begin to speak to yourself in the words you would say to comfort a frightened child. By not giving over your power to your fear, you are freed to move forward at whatever pace suites you.

Will it come back? There is no way of knowing. Yet you can be present in the moments of your life, living each day as fully as you can. Being in the present doesn't happen tomorrow, nor does it exist in yesterday. Circumstances change; situations change; we change. You really can't know what you'll do unless or until "it" does come back. Your personal choice may not be evident until you are presented with a specific situation. What is always true is that you get to decide based on what is right for you. The importance of giving yourself this deeply personal choice is highlighted in the question "What will I do if it comes back?" It may not be a choice that you will ever need to make and regardless, you probably can't really make until you have to. And . . . you may never have to make that choice.

> "At age seventy-six I am now twelve years past my first bout with cancer and it's been four years since my second. . . . I don't think I have any concerns that I did not have before. I am acutely aware of our built-in obsolescence and limited shelf life on this planet."
>
> **—Len, cancer survivor**

> "It's important to eat right, exercise, and see your doctor for follow-up visits, but please understand that these measures cannot keep cancer from recurring. Many

cancer patients blame themselves for missing a doctor visit, not eating right, or post-poning a CT scan for a family vacation. But even if you do everything just right, the cancer still might come back."

—American Cancer Society, *Living with Uncertainty*[7]

GRATITUDE

"You're not ever finished. There's just a sense that this phase is over."

—Margie, cancer survivor

A friend said to me, "You dodged a bullet." This is a powerful reminder that in surviving, you are given another chance at life. Gratitude for this opportunity—this reprieve—can begin to fill in the blank after the question, "Will it come back?" Gratitude opens the doors and windows that fear snaps shut. You can learn to open to possibilities. You have an opportunity to grow beyond old habits, stale ideas and stories, and outworn fantasies of who you believe you are and the life you think you *should* be living. This can be like the open road, the sea in front of you with no sight of land for miles, the Montana skies. The discovery of freedom in the midst of facing illness creates a powerful place within the soul. It's like getting in the car and taking off without looking back, heading for a place where you have always wanted to go but never dared to dream it possible. What do you need to leave behind? What do you need to unpack? What will you choose to take with you?

Another chance, the bullet missed its mark. This gratitude does not come easily. It has as its price authentic gratitude; deep gratitude from the heart usually does. Gratitude for each day, for the hope of seeing your children grow up, the sun as it sparkles on water, the smell of jasmine on a warm day; the light of gratitude is the gift of darkness' struggle. Gratitude can carry you over rocks and across flooded streams. It may show you the whys and wherefores of being alive in each moment. You've been given another chance.

In the depth of your hopes and desires
lies your silent knowledge of the beyond;
And like seeds dreaming beneath the snow
your heart dreams of spring.
—Kahlil Gibran, "On Death"[8]

"It ain't over 'til it's over"
—Yogi Berra[9]

WORKBOOK SECTION: HOW TO DEAL WITH FEAR

We've acknowledged that your fear of cancer recurrence is normal, but now it's time to review some ways to work with that fear so you don't remain frozen with it. After recognizing that fear exists in response to a life-threatening illness, you can move forward by bringing respectful attention, curiosity, and compassion to your fright. This workbook section is designed to help you examine and understand your fear so that you feel more emotionally in charge. You can use your fear to have a better understanding of your challenges, which can then make it easier for you to make more conscious choices. This way of reflection suggests that a deep learning can come from understanding and facing your fears and helps you to feel empowered.

How Do You Experience Your Fear?

1. What brings up your fears of a cancer recurrence? How do those fears arise within you?

2. What are the sensations you notice in your body when you feel afraid?

3. What kind of thoughts race through your mind when you are in a state of fear?

4. Describe your experience with fear. For example, do you freeze or become agitated? Does your fear hide beneath anger or other emotions?

5. What stories does your fear tell you about cancer?

Ways to Deal with Your Fear

Now that you've spent some time identifying and understanding your fear, here are some practices that can help you regulate your fear reactions. Remember that these are merely tools that help you feel more in charge. They are not meant to deny the normal feelings of fear that the theme of cancer recurrence brings up but are offered to you as a way to take back the power you give to fear. These suggestions help you to face down the bogeyman of fear:

1. In the previous section you were asked about when you find yourself telling a story about cancer recurrence. One way to deal with these stories is to stop and realize that it's only your imagination making up a scary story that isn't true and then bring yourself into the present moment. Remind yourself that it is a story you don't need to create. You can write your own story.

2. Greet your fear with a neutral attitude: "Oh, fear, hello."

3. Tell your fear that it is welcome and ask it to show you the lessons you are learning from it. What lessons is your fear teaching you?

4. Have a conversation with your fear. What is it saying to you? What do you say back to your fear?

5. If your fear remains persistent and won't leave you alone, get tough with it. Tell your fear, in no uncertain terms, to go away. Treat your fear the same way you would if someone was bullying you: Stand up and send it away. Think of a strong statement to confront your fear and write it down now.

6. Talk to someone. Fears have a way of getting huge when we are alone with them. You can banish some of those scary monsters if you express your fears to another person.

Transforming Fear into Gratitude

By learning to face your fear of cancer recurrence, you become open to new possibilities. Letting go of your fears to simply be in the present moment with what is opens up a place to recognize what you are grateful for. Gratitude does not have to be grand. It can be found not only in our joys but also in our sorrows. You can use these questions to open up to your feelings of gratitude.

1. What are you grateful for today?

2. What are you grateful for in your life?

3. Who are you grateful for?

4. How are you grateful for yourself?

5. Write a note of gratitude about your healing from cancer.

NOTES

1. Stanley Plumly, "Cancer," in *Orphan Hours* (New York: W. W. Norton, 2012), 26–27. Used by permission of W. W. Norton & Company, Inc. © 2012 by Stanley Plumly.

2. Irvin. D. Yalom, *Staring at the Sun: Overcoming the Terror of Death* (San Francisco: Jossey-Bass, 2009), 11. Used by permission of John Wiley & Sons, Inc. © 2008, 2009 by Irvin D. Yalom.

3. American Cancer Society, *Living with Uncertainty: The Fear of Cancer Recurrence,* last revised June 19, 2013, www.cancer.org/acs/groups/cid/documents/webcontent/002014-pdf.pdf, p. 3.

4. American Cancer Society, *Living with Uncertainty*, 2.

5. *50/50*, directed by Jonathan Levine (2011; Santa Monica, CA: Summit Entertainment). Used by permission of Summit Entertainment, LLC.

6. American Cancer Society, *Living with Uncertainty*, 8.

7. American Cancer Society, *Living with Uncertainty*, 4.

8. Kahlil Gibran, "On Death," in *The Prophet* (New York: Knopf, 1973), 80. Used by permission of Alfred A. Knopf, an imprint of the Knopf Doubleday Publishing Group, a division of Penguin Random House LLC. All rights reserved. © 1923 by Kahlil Gibran and renewed 1951 by Administrators C. T. A. of Kahlil Gibran Estate, and Mary G. Gibran.

9. Yogi Berra, *The Yogi Book* (New York: Workman, 2010), 13. Used by permission of Workman Publishing Co., Inc., New York. © 1998, 2019 by L.T. D. Enterprises.

DEALING WITH UNCERTAINTY

STEERING THROUGH DARKNESS WITH NO STARS

5

It is touch I go by,
the boat like a hand feeling
through shoals and among
dead trees, over the boulders
lifting unseen, layer
on layer on drowned time falling away.
This is how I learned to steer
through darkness with no stars.
To be lost is only a failure of memory.
—Margaret Atwood, "A Boat"[1]

LIVING WITH UNCERTAINTY IS ONE OF THE major concerns we face as cancer survivors. I've seen this theme appear on every survey given to cancer patients and listened to survivors talk about it in therapy sessions, group discussions, and casual conversation. Sometimes it is named, but often uncertainty comes disguised as obsessive fear or shows up in searches for some kind of guarantee that illness will not return. Our thoughts and feelings around uncertainty can't be addressed by an electronic slide presentation, a diet, or an exercise program. Exploring the truth of uncertainty is a deeply personal process. Learning to live with uncertainty may be your greatest challenge and your most profound opportunity after drawing the short straw of cancer.

"Cancer survivors probably live with more uncertainty than people who deal with other kinds of illness. This may be because cancer is generally difficult to treat, and there is a good chance that it will recur."
—Hester Hill Schnipper, LICSW, Oncology Social Work Chief at Beth Israel Deaconess Medical Center in Boston[2]

Accepting uncertainty creates freedom. Yet we demonize uncertainty; we think of it as something that should go away quietly and leave us alone. We swear and scream at it and run away from it because we're frightened by what we don't know and what we can't control. But the creature of uncertainty, when ignored, will search for you in your dreams and haunt you in the ruminating obsessions of your days. Banished from your consciousness, fear returns from your unconscious depths as a monster that creates bigger and scarier stories than you need to carry around within you. Facing the "monster under the bed" of uncertainty and letting go of scary stories to explore your own authentic relationship with whatever comes through the doors and windows of your consciousness brings you aliveness and an opportunity to engage with what is real in your life. Being willing to meet and explore the challenges of uncertainty after cancer by exploring who you are now in your life allows a space for personal transformation.

> "The only moment we know for sure that we have survived cancer is the moment we die of something else."
> **—Denise, cancer survivor**

In reality, you live with a great absence of certainty. You weren't born with a warranty or guarantee that you could control the world around you. Yet we are taught from an early age to know the *right* answers and encouraged to plan for what we are told will be a secure future. A cancer diagnosis is a startling reminder of just how insecure we really do feel about our futures. The plans we had on our to-do lists change drastically as we learn how to negotiate the first phase of dealing with diagnosis and the decisions that face us at this time.

THE FIRST PHASE OF UNCERTAINTY: AM I GOING TO MAKE IT?

Moving into the first phase of dealing with cancer involves to-do lists. Feeling shocked and chaotic, you need to make decisions and learn about various treatment options, which is confusing and scary. This all takes place while in a state of disbelief that this is really happening to you. Even as you are actively choosing the direction you will take, you're thinking, "Uh, oh. Am I going to make it? What kind of treatment will I have? What will the treatments be like? Can I work? Can I continue going to school? What will my friends think? How will I care for my kids? Will I lose my hair? Am I going to be an invalid?" You are busy trying to figure out what to do to stay alive.

> "The uncertainty between finding cancer and the lab results after the surgery were the most intense for me."
> **—Doreen, cancer survivor**

Crisis can create certainty. When we make choices based on an active treatment plan, we feel a sense of power. We're doing something about the cancer. There are clear directions to follow. After treatment begins, we start to understand what the experience is like for us. We begin to figure out how to handle this part of our lives one day at a time. The routine of treatment becomes familiar. Often we feel miserably ill and weak from the intensity of the treatment we are receiving. As horrific as it can be, we have a plan of action. The treatment phase of cancer provides structure as well as constant contact with your providers. And then, you're done . . .

> "I recall double- or triple-checking with nurses and doctors as to when they wanted to see me again, whether that was really the right time, had they forgotten something? My cancer came out of the blue, totally by surprise. I was young. I thought I was healthy with no prior history of cancer. It snuck up on me once. Wasn't there someone who'd be able to prevent that from happening again?"
> **—Julie, cancer survivor**

THE SECOND PHASE OF UNCERTAINTY: AM I ALLOWED TO BE HOPEFUL?

Swiss philosopher and poet Henri Frederic Amiel said, "Uncertainty is the refuge of hope."[3] Hope can be a true companion and a troublemaker. We need hope like we need companionship. But hope can also be tyrannical and hold you hostage with the pretense of control and certainty. How do you know your hope is real? There is no measure, no numerical scale, so hope becomes another member of the family of uncertainty. The companionship of hope gets you up in the morning and sends you off into another day. It's a good day if you lay down that night with the arms of hope around you.

The smoldering embers of uncertainty burst into flames when treatment ends. The waiting game begins and you might want to stay on the bench waiting for the bus, never catching the next ride, paralyzed with a kind of numbing fearfulness that closes your eyes and ears to what is happening all around you. You don't know what to do or where to go. You feel lost. You can start to miss living your life.

> "Everybody's got something. In the end, what choice does one have but to understand that truth, to really take it in, and then shop for groceries, get a haircut; do one's work, get on with the business of life. That's the hope anyway."
> —**David Rakoff**, *Half Empty*[4]

Getting on with the business of your life is not always so easy. You thought you were headed for Denver and next thing you know, you're in Detroit. You hold onto the belief that your life is certain; that you can know what will happen around the next bend. Because we believe that we can actually control things, we want things to be certain; we want to know what will happen. Why is it so tempting to dwell in the land of what we believe to be certain when it can lead to boredom and a deadened sense of negatively scripted reality? We stay here despite how bleak it may feel, largely because it is familiar to us. Yet allowing the mystery of uncertainty to touch you can lead to unexpected chances, creating adventures and events you may never have dreamed possible. It's not static or predictable, it's a way to feel more alive.

Uncertainty creates curiosity. Remember how, as a child, the summer days seemed to stretch on endlessly? You experienced joy in the small discoveries of grasshoppers or newfound places in the woods. You noticed the clouds blowing by, changing shape into animals or faces. Recapture that childlike innocence, which trusts that the next moment will arrive as it will.

Each moment does arrive as it will. The sooner we overcome our delusions of control, the more spontaneous and joyful we become. Being willing to accept the paradox that letting go of certainty may actually lead to a deeper sense of relief and well-being helps you to move forward. You learn that while you aren't in control, you do have choices.

> "As human beings, not only do we seek resolution, but we also feel that we deserve resolution. However, not only do we not deserve resolution, we suffer from resolution. We don't deserve resolution; we deserve something better than that. We deserve our birthright, which is the middle way, an open state of mind that can relax with paradox and ambiguity."
> —**Pema Chödrön**, *When Things Fall Apart*[5]

Greeting uncertainty with an open mind moves you off the bench and on to the next bus. You don't know your destination. You can know and experience how having an open mind allows for movement. It allows you to be lighter and more flexible. It is interesting to think of getting to know ambiguity as a way to relax into this lightness. Imagine sitting on that bus, looking out the window, and noticing the landscape you are passing through. It is unfamiliar and may be gray and depressing, yet it's in continual movement. Next you might find yourself staring out on a beautiful field of sunflowers, their heads raised to take in a luminous golden sun. The bus continues and you notice the trees, buildings, people, the moon, and stars. They all appear and then fade away. You still have no clue where you are, but you relax into your seat and enjoy the scenery. You let yourself surrender to the moments of your life without the need to judge or control what is occurring.

> "Surrender brought me to my knees and just where I needed to be to restore my faith in life."
> —**Barbara, cancer survivor**

IT'S NOT FAIR

Holding on to the belief that life is fair is another way to avoid the truth of uncertainty. Years ago I was in a local market and overheard a conversation between a mother and her little boy. The boy was angling for something he wanted and quite persistent in his requests. Mom held her ground, firmly stating no. He wailed, "This is not fair!" She slowly turned to him, bent down, looked him square in the eyes, and said, "Sweetie, this is about as fair as it's going to get." None of us is given a promise of fairness, and while it is compelling to wail, "It's not fair" at cancer, this response is just another way to stay stuck on the bench.

Embedded in the attachment to fairness is the illusion that being good will somehow ensure that we will get what we want or, at the very least, we'll be rescued from disaster. If I exercise, eat right, and keep a positive outlook on life, I won't get cancer and certainly I won't get it again. Facing the letting go of our childhood belief in fairness is one of the most difficult tasks of growing up. Facing our own mortality and the lack of control around that is one of the most difficult tasks of adulthood. No wonder we all have some fantasy of being Peter Pan and flying off to Neverland. If I never grow up, does it mean I won't die? Fairness implies that there are standards that are universally obeyed, especially when one plays by the rules. As children we are taught that when we are good, we get what we want, and when we are bad, we don't. The land of magical thinking is a delightful place and it's compelling to live there for eternity. The major impact of a cancer diagnosis can really seem unfair if we've played by the rules and still get sick. Again, it's difficult to grasp that we just don't have that much control over what happens to us but to linger in the mythology of fairness only keeps us stuck.

> "I wanted a perfect ending. Now I learned, the hard way, that some poems don't rhyme, and some stories don't have a clear beginning, middle and end. Life is about not knowing, having to change, taking the moment and making the best of it, without knowing what's going to happen next. Delicious Ambiguity."
> —**Gilda Radner,** *It's Always Something*[6]

HOW TELLING YOUR STORY HELPS

Delicious ambiguity, a curious and open mind, and learning to steer through darkness with no stars, are all facets of living with uncertainty.

In the exploration and expression of your survivor story, you become an integral part of the process of moving through and beyond cancer. This can provide you with a structure if you are a person living with cancer. If you feel connected and comfortable with your treatment team, you may choose to share your story as an adjunct to the traditional survivor care plan in your medical records. If this is an option, your medical team may be able to help you focus on identifying your emotional needs and then make appropriate referrals. If you work with a hospital social worker with whom you have a good relationship, then that professional can help you put together the resources you will need whether you live with cancer or have moved beyond the treatment phase of cancer. These resources may include financial as well as social services information. You may choose to work with a psychotherapist to help you explore the thoughts and feelings that will arise as you reflect on the questions of your survivorship.

It is important to acknowledge the impact that cancer has on everyone involved. As defined in this book, survivors include the patients, partners, families, and friends. Each group has specific needs, so the story templates are separated according to those categories. Partners, family members, and friends often feel excluded, helpless, guilty, and unsure about how to express their own feelings and needs. Parents of survivors are affected because they have to cope with the illness and possible death of their child all the while needing to provide strength and hope throughout the process. They certainly need to have someone to turn to, to collapse into when they have a moment for their own reflection.

> "I remember sitting there completely unconcerned for the worst as the doctor spoke about looking at the X-rays. Michele excused herself for a moment. I looked at the doctor and simply asked what he thought it was. Then he said those words that I think most people would be devastated to hear when relating to a loved one: 'She has cancer.' Still, today, as I write these words and relive the moment, tears come to my eyes."
> **—Debbie, mother**

I have created a separate story workbook section for young cancer survivors as their concerns are different. The difficulties of this group are just beginning to be recognized. They are at the beginning of creating their lives when they face the possibility that the life they are planning might not happen. Older survivors, by contrast, sometimes face a bias: "You've lived your life, so just be quiet and grateful and go away." Cancer is many diseases and treatments vary, so life with and after cancer is unique to each individual. My hope is that the templates provided in this book are helpful no matter who you are or what you're facing, and that they'll offer you an avenue for insight as well as an opportunity for clarity and personal growth.

All the templates are designed to share with others. If you are a cancer patient who has young children, you could use the material as a way to talk with your children and help them understand their own feelings about having a parent who has survived cancer. Partners can find ways to help one another understand their experience by sharing their stories. The same is true for friends, family members, and colleagues.

Children who survive or are living with cancer need help understanding their experiences. The template for young children is created as an interview with the possibility of using art and toys as vehicles for nonverbal expression. It is important to meet the child as a person who has different ways of working with thoughts and feelings.

You didn't put having cancer on your to-do list. You can tell your story and create a thoughtful memoir that gives you a map that you have crafted to guide you through these unchartered waters. Since you're still around, you might as well take part in your life, and create your stories regardless of whether they have a clear beginning, middle, or end. Your changing story becomes the boat that holds you as you learn to steer through the waters of uncertainty in both darkness and light until you find yourself where you are now. In the end, it's really all you can count on. In the open space of the awareness, you keep falling forward from one moment to the next, learning to live with uncertainty as you go.

> *We've never heard about the day we were conceived*
> *Nor the doctor who helped us to be born,*
> *Nor that blind old man who decides when we will die*
> *It's hard to understand why the sun rises,*
> *And why our children are mostly fond of us,*
> *And why the wind blows the curtains in the afternoon.*
> **—Robert Bly,** "The Blind Old Man"[7]

WORKBOOK SECTION: TELL YOUR STORY

After finishing treatment for cancer, many of us still feel unfinished with what has just happened to us. We feel a need to be able to speak about our experiences so that we can better understand and begin to integrate them into our lives as we move forward. My healthcare providers generally did not check in with me after treatment, and I never received a survivor care plan that focused on my emotional experiences. I know that my experience is common, and that many of you are also left feeling frustrated, frightened, and lost in post-treatment.

The questions in this workbook section are designed to help you reflect on your experience with having cancer. There aren't any right or wrong answers. I hope you can use this workbook as a way to give yourself a place for needed reflection. Please give yourself time and space to be with these narrative questions. And if you feel it would be helpful, share what you discover with your partner, your families, and your friends. If you have a good relationship with your healthcare team, you may choose to share your reflections with them as well.

1. It all began when:

2. How are you? What would you like to talk about?

3. What was it like when you first heard that you had cancer?

4. How was your experience of being in treatment for cancer?

5. How have things been going for you since you finished treatment? Describe your experience of finishing treatment for cancer. Notice what stands out for you. What was most helpful and what was least helpful?

6. Describe your experience if you are someone who is living with cancer. What is most helpful and what is least helpful for you as you continue to negotiate your way through treatment?

7. What feelings and concerns about your cancer diagnosis do you feel that you carry within you?

8. What really scares you? (Write your experience.)

9. What are your concerns regarding your physical health? For example, do you have fatigue, pain, weight issues, or sleep difficulties? How do you feel about addressing these with your doctors?

10. Do you feel listened to by others? Or do you worry that you are being a burden when you talk about your concerns?

11. Do you have financial concerns?

12. How would you say that your life changed after completion of treatment for cancer?

13. What would you say about how your life has changed if you are someone who is living with cancer?

14. Are you hopeful? What do you hope for in your life?

15. What kind of changes have you experienced in your relationships with your partner, family members, and friends?

16. Do you have concerns about sexuality and intimate relationships?

17. When do you feel worried and scared?

18. What makes you feel relaxed and happy?

19. How do you feel changed by your experience of cancer?

20. What matters to you? (Write what comes to you.)

21. When did you feel like a survivor? Or do you?

22. What could have been emotionally supportive after finishing treatment?

23. What is emotionally supportive if you are living with cancer?

24. If you could do whatever you wanted, you would:

After you have spent some time with these questions, reflecting on what thoughts and feelings arise, move on to the next exercise in this workbook section, which is divided into two parts: Short-Term Intentions and Long-Term Intentions. Short-term intentions cover a period from the present to approximately eighteen months and help you focus on who you are now in your life. Long-term intentions aid you in setting intentions for the future based on what you deeply value in the bigger picture of your life. Long-term intentions may take years to bring to fruition.

The exploration into your intentions weaves the topic of quality of life into your story template. As a framework, I use the quality of life definition from the University of Toronto Quality of Life Research Unit: Quality of life is "the degree to which a person enjoys the important possibilities of his or her life. Possibilities result from the opportunities and limitations each person has in [his or her] life and reflect the interaction of personal and environmental factors." Three major life domains are identified: being, belonging, and becoming.[8]

Please note that your definition of quality of life is uniquely your own and extremely personal, so I encourage you to spend time exploring exactly what quality of life means to you.

Think of this as a narrative. Imagine that you are being asked the questions, and then respond as if you were having a dialogue with another person. You may want to imagine speaking to your oncologist, surgeon, or radiologist. You might envision a friend, therapist, or spiritual advisor. Or you may feel comfortable having this dialogue with yourself. Don't worry about right or wrong answers, because they don't exist. You may want to update this story template from time to time as you move forward in your life and your needs change.

Exercise: Short-Term Intentions

Short-term intentions can take the pressure off of thinking that you need to know what you want in the long term before you take stock of where you are in the present moment. Slow down and release the pressure of moving beyond where you are now in your life. This is likely still a time for recovery and rejuvenation. Initially, short-term intentions may look like reading a book, taking a bath, having a cup of tea, taking a walk, or watching a movie. Intentions aren't difficult and often don't require a lot of planning. After you've gotten into a rhythm with them, then you can start to look twelve to eighteen months in the future.

MY SHORT-TERM INTENTIONS:

Exercise: Long-Term Intentions

Long-term intentions require self-inquiry into what you value and what is important to you in the bigger picture of your life. A good question to ask yourself when contemplating your long-term intentions is: "*What really matters to me?*" Sitting with this question and watching what emerges can lead you to a place of self-discovery, which allows you to thoughtfully choose your life path based on who you are now. Long-term intentions may look like work or career interests, creative pursuits, and relationships and intimacy with others as well as within yourself. This search is not necessarily motivated by external circumstances or materialistic pursuits, but it can be. It is important to value the realistic aspects of long-term intentions but not get caught up in how productive or practical they *should* be. Allow for the voice of your innermost wants and dreams to be heard, which means that you don't have to settle for less than what you really believe to be possible for yourself. Both interior and exterior personal worlds are a part of this exploration. Take time and allow yourself to be with your thoughts and feelings without the need to create goals and plans before you are sure of what really does matter to you. It's easy to get caught up in measuring success by the standards of family pressures or societal bias. We can all fall into the trap of wanting to look good to others rather than choosing the right path for ourselves. I once worked with a woman who achieved a high level of corporate success and left it all happily behind to train guide dogs. Colleagues are constantly after me to raise my fees, yet I purposely have kept them lower than average because I want to cultivate a diverse and creative client base in my private practice. What pleases you is up to *you*.

MY LONG-TERM INTENTIONS:

Tell Your Story (for Young Survivors)

This was probably the last thing you expected at this stage of your life, right? You're just starting out, whether you're still in school, early in your career, or starting a family. The trajectory of your life got rerouted, and it can be tough to watch your peers moving on with their plans while you are struggling with surviving a cancer diagnosis. And yet, your needs and concerns differ from others with cancer diagnoses who are older than you. The questions that are provided for your group of survivors are written with this perspective in mind.

After finishing treatment for cancer, you may still feel unfinished with what has just happened to you. As a younger cancer survivor, you may feel even more isolated. You might want to speak about your experience so that you can better understand and begin to integrate it into your life as you move forward. The questions in this workbook section are designed to help you reflect on your experience with cancer. There aren't any right or wrong answers. I hope you can use this workbook as a way to give yourself a place for needed reflection. Give yourself time and space to be with these narrative questions. And if you feel it would be helpful, share what you discover with your partner, families, or friends. If you are comfortable, you may also choose to share your reflections with your healthcare team.

1. How did it all begin for you?

2. How are you?

3. What do you want to talk about? Do you feel like people give you the space to talk about your experience?

4. How is your family? Are they anxious about you? Dealing with my family around my cancer has been . . . (write your thoughts and feelings)

5. How's it going in school? Have there been cognitive changes that affect your work?

6. How do you feel that your experience with cancer is affecting your job and career path? What are your concerns?

7. How's it going with your friends and your social network? Do you feel like you fit in? Do the people around you get what you're going through?

8. Do you sometimes feel more mature than your peer group? How does that show up and what does it feel like to you?

9. Do you feel understood? Who can you talk to?

10. What are your concerns about sexuality? Are you concerned with fertility challenges? Do you feel comfortable talking about these concerns and issues? How and when do you decide to bring them up?

11. What's it like to deal with your physical changes and challenges, such as fatigue, scarring, losses, and other ways in which your body has been affected by cancer and treatments? How does this affect your self-image?

12. What's it like to be at a place in your life where you may need to depend more on your family when you want to become more independent and start your own life?

13. What happens when you have been out on your own and need to return to get the help and support you need?

14. What are your biggest worries and fears?

15. What makes you happy and relaxed?

16. How do you feel changed by your experience?

SURVIVING THE STORM

17. I really wish I . . . (write your thoughts and feelings)

18. When did you feel like a survivor? Or do you?

19. If you are someone who is living with cancer, what is your experience?

At this point, it may be useful to acknowledge what it may be like to make a plan for the future while facing a future that may at the same time seem so uncertain. With so much of life ahead of you, it might seem scary or even stupid to look too far into an uncertain future. This is not what you expected at this stage of your life. While that is tough, I encourage you to take the risk of focusing on your short-term as well as long-term intentions. Letting go of your worry about the consequences *may* actually be the best thing you do for yourself.

After you have spent some time with the questions in the template, reflecting on what thoughts and feelings arise, move on to the two exercises that follow: Short-term Intentions and Long-term Intentions. Short-term intentions cover a period from the present to approximately eighteen months and help you focus on who you are now in your life. Long-term intentions aid you in making plans for the future based on what you deeply value in the bigger picture of your life. Think of this as a narrative. Imagine that you are being asked the questions and then respond as if you were having a dialogue with another person. You may want to imagine speaking to your oncologist, surgeon, or radiologist. You might envision a friend, therapist, or spiritual advisor. Or you may feel comfortable having this dialogue with yourself. Don't worry about right or wrong answers, because they don't exist. You may want to redo this exercise from time to time as you move forward in your life and your needs change.

Exercise: Short-Term Intentions

Short-term intentions can take the pressure off of thinking that you need to know what you want in the long term before you take stock of where you are in the present moment. Slow down and release the pressure of moving beyond where you are now in your life. This is likely still a time for recovery and rejuvenation. Initially, short-term intentions may look like reading a book, taking a bath, having a cup of tea, taking a walk, or watching a movie. They aren't difficult and often don't require a lot of planning. You may then move on to short-term intentions that look forward twelve to eighteen months. This is when you feel stronger and more able to focus. These intentions may involve work, relationships, creative projects, and things that may take some planning. However, remember that these intentions aren't forever, are flexible and, in that way, doable.

MY SHORT-TERM INTENTIONS:

Exercise: Long-Term Intentions

Long-term intentions require self-inquiry into what you value and what is important to you in the bigger picture of your life. A good question to ask yourself is: "What really matters to me?" Sitting with this question and watching what emerges can lead you to a place of self-discovery that allows you to thoughtfully choose your life path based on who you are now. Long-term intentions may look like work or career interests, creative pursuits, and relationships and intimacy with others as well as within yourself. This search is not necessarily motivated by external circumstances or materialistic pursuits, yet both of these areas may be included. It is important to value the realistic aspects of long-term intentions but not get caught on how productive or practical they *should* be so as to allow for the voice of your innermost wants and dreams to be heard. In essence, do not settle for less than what you really believe to be possible for yourself. Both interior and exterior personal worlds are a part of this exploration. Take time and allow yourself to be with your thoughts and feelings without the need to create goals and plans before you are sure of what really does matter to you.

It's easy to get caught up in measuring success by the standards of family pressure or societal bias. We can all fall into the trap of "looking good" to others rather than choosing the right path for ourselves. I once worked with a woman who achieved a high level of corporate success and left it all happily behind to train guide dogs. Colleagues are constantly after me to raise my fees, yet I purposely have kept them lower than average, which has created a diverse and creative client base in my private practice. What pleases you is up to *you*.

MY LONG-TERM INTENTIONS:

NOTES

1. Margaret Atwood, "A Boat," in *Selected Poems II: Poems Selected and New, 1976-1986* (Boston: Houghton Mifflin, 1987), 120. Used by permission of Houghton Mifflin Harcourt Publishing Company. All rights reserved. © 1987 by Margaret Atwood.

2. LiveStrong Foundation, *Fear of Recurrence*, 2011, www.fredhutch.org/content/dam/public/ Treatment-Suport/survivorship/Healthy-Links/Fear%20of%20Recurrence.pdf, p. 1

3. Henri Frederic Amiel, BrainyQuote.com, Xplore Inc, 2016, www.brainyquote.com/quotes/ quotes/h/henrifrede165136.html, accessed October 4, 2016.

4. David Rakoff, *Half Empty* (New York: Doubleday, 2010), 224. Used by permission of Irene Skolnick Literary Agency as agent for the author and Doubleday, an imprint of the Knopf Doubleday Publishing Group, a division of Penguin Random House LLC. All rights reserved. Any third party use of this material outside of this publication is prohibited. Interested parties must apply directly to Penguin Random House LLC for permission. © 2010, 2011 by David Rakoff.

5. Pema Chödrön, *When Things Fall Apart: Heart Advice for Difficult Times* (Boulder, CO: Shambhala, 1997), 52. Used by permission of The Permissions Company, Inc. on behalf of Shambhala Publications Inc., Boulder, Colorado, www.shambhala.com. © 1997 by Pema Chödrön.

6. Gilda Radner, *It's Always Something* (New York: Simon & Schuster, 1989), 254. Used by permission of Simon and Schuster, Inc. All rights reserved. © 1989 by Gilda Radner.

7. Robert Bly, "The Blind Old Man," in Talking into the Ear of a Donkey (New York: W. W. Norton, 2011), 29. Used by permission of Georges Borchardt Inc., for Robert Bly and W.W. Norton & Company, Inc. © 2010, 2011 by Robert Bly.

8. "Quality of Life Model," Quality of Life Research Unit, University of Toronto, Ontario, accessed September 29, 2016, http://sites.utoronto.ca/qol/qol_model.htm.

WHAT DO I DO? WHAT DO I SAY? WHAT ABOUT ME?

6

PARTNERS, FAMILIES, AND FRIENDS AS SURVIVORS

Her breast cancer, she said,
had metastasized to her liver;
she was going to die, and
soon. She said it made her
sad. I didn't know her well.
We were co-workers and
I liked her, but
what do you say when someone
actually answers the question
how are you?
with the unvarnished truth:
Not well, *she said.* I haven't
long to live. *And should I*
have said Oh you will! *Should I*
have smoothed it over
with the syrup of nervousness,
or done what I did
which was to
talk about terror and anger,
the unfairness and the lie,
to take the truth the truth at face value?
No, she was just sad, *she said,*
She had her faith, *she said,*
and started to cry. And only then
did I see what she needed from me
was miracle, a simple belief
in miracle, and if that was varnish,
well, it would bring the grain
of the truth out, would save it
from wear and weather.
It would make the truth
almost shine.

—Ronald Wallace, "The Truth"[1]

> " . . . it was a big "oh shit" moment."
> —**Wilma**, learning that a close friend had cancer

> "All through treatment, I longed for a place where I belonged. Nothing felt quite right and maybe that was just because of the helplessness of the situation. I mostly felt like an outsider during the process, although I was intimately involved with everything that was happening—every procedure, every decision along the way. I guess I wanted to be able to tell someone how I felt, that I was terrified beyond words, that I was overwhelmed with all the issues of my immediate family. I was falling apart internally but it seemed like there was no one who was able to help me."
> —**Jill**, daughter

LIFE IS FOREVER CHANGED FOR THOSE OF YOU affected by the cancer diagnosis of someone you love. You may find yourself in the role of caregiver, in addition to all the other roles you have in your life. You may feel forgotten in the wake of the chaos of illness. Your time and energy can be called upon in ways you could not have foreseen. Life has suddenly taken a sharp turn. Maybe you feel guilty about having feelings of your own and don't feel as if you have anyone you can talk with about what you're going through. Don't let your suffering and heartache remain silent. Your stories are also important and need to be told.

Those of you in relationship with the patient are also survivors. In just a moment, a partner, friend, daughter, or mother may take on a new role: cancer caregiver. A sibling's daily experience may be altered significantly. A child senses something is very wrong with a parent but has no way to express his or her feelings. Friends, who can be closer than family members, are deeply affected, uncertain about how to be helpful, and sometimes get left behind in the upheaval. All too often the troubles and intense emotional responses of those affected by cancer remain unacknowledged. The level of metamorphosis in a relationship that ensues after a diagnosis is extreme. It's a transformation with a hazardous component that can cause people to lapse into a confused silence and become mute. And yet they are also called upon to respond to the life-threatening illness of someone they love.

If you are helping someone get through cancer treatment, you are a caregiver, and you have your own story to tell. Recently, there has been increased awareness about the need to support caregivers, particularly when it comes to the adjustments and difficulties surrounding survivorship in those first months and years after the end of treatment. Balancing your own life with those you care for becomes a challenge. It's not easy to do, particularly without support.

> "PTSD can also affect caregivers. Learning that a loved one has cancer, seeing a loved one in pain, and experiencing a medical emergency are traumatic events. And they may contribute to the development of PTSD symptoms during treatment or years after the person has survived the cancer. One study found that nearly 20% of families with teenaged survivors of childhood cancer had a parent who was experiencing PTSD. Research also shows that it is extremely common for parents of children receiving cancer treatment to develop stress-related symptoms."
> —**Cancer.Net**, "PTSD and Caregivers"[2]

The ongoing stress on those of you who are caregivers can cause emotional and physical difficulties that go unnoticed. While it has become somewhat routine to use a distress screening form for the patient who has been diagnosed with cancer, it is rarely something that is given to the caregiver. Have you had much experience with being asked about your distress or well-being? Do you feel like people ask you how you are doing? Your thoughts and feelings are equally valuable, as you have been involved in most of the events and encounters with not only the patient but the patient's healthcare team. Integrated healthcare includes everyone who is involved in the trauma of life-threatening illness and it is vital to provide distress screening for *all* of you. This may not necessarily be a form that you fill out in the provider's office or a hospital, but it is important that you have outlets for the expression of your concerns. Following up with what has emerged from a distress survey, or having a conversation about it, is also essential. Otherwise, you are left with the awareness of your struggles with no one to talk to, no possible resolution, and the feeling that you have nowhere to go for help.

You may have concerns about getting help for yourself as the caregiver, concerns about time and space for your own needs, and worry and pressure about being away from the patient—your loved one—for too long. Changes in the roles and interpersonal dynamics and issues of control are not unusual visitors for those of you in relationship with someone who has cancer. You've had the strenuous task of taking care of someone on multiple levels while balancing numerous other aspects of your life. These difficulties don't negate the deeply gratifying and meaningful moments of caring for someone, but just acknowledge the complexity of your role.

While some people facing a life-threatening situation may find a newfound clarity about what really matters to them, for others communication can become strained, and one or both people can become withdrawn. Having an outlet for conversation about what's happening helps both parties, and if they're willing, new possibilities of intimacy can result. Realizing that it is important not to take someone for granted may bring a new level of connection and honesty that expresses a genuine love and allows room for difficult issues. There's a sense of urgency that comes from facing a life-threatening illness with another person that provides an opportunity for a meaningful dialogue reaching beyond the boundaries of what you may have previously allowed in your relationship. Realizing that time is precious underlies this sense of urgency and meaning, and it can move you into a stronger intimacy with one another. When you are in touch with the ephemeral nature of your life, you are free to be open and to take chances in your relationship. Letting go of old constraints and connecting in this way might even lead to the adoption of a risk-embracing kind of attitude that helps the relationship grow more alive.

Yet your role as a caregiver doesn't always feel meaningful. Again, there are so many aspects of all that you are going through that you may sometimes feel confused about who you are anymore. The outpouring of feelings you have around being a caregiver, on top of the suffering you are witnessing, runs deep and jagged. Within your heart, you may feel daunted by the task before you, while at the same time you carry the expectation that you should rise above your own experience. You may struggle with feelings of helplessness as you scramble to figure out what to say and what to do. You're no doubt frightened and exhausted. And, perhaps most difficult of all, you feel alone.

You are an important and growing group in survivorship, and you, too, are desperately in need of being heard. This chapter and its workbook section are designed to give you the attention and space you need to begin to address your concerns.

> "Humankind has not woven the web of life. We are but one thread within it. Whatever we do to the web, we do to ourselves. All things are bound together. All things connect."
> **—Chief Seattle**[3]

WHAT IT MEANS TO BE A CAREGIVER

Giving care can include a number of services. You may be giving hands-on care by bathing and feeding someone. You may be taking your loved one to doctor's appointments, sitting with him or her in the treatment room, or cooking meals and cleaning. It is likely that your life has gotten more complicated and that your personal time has become severely compromised. Care can also include helping someone cope with their feelings and listening to their emotional distress. Although few of the caregivers I've spoken with verbalized it, the expectations and pressure to be giving at all times is intense and can seriously intrude on the needs of the caregiver. It is difficult to express these kinds of emotions and feelings of pressure and to speak of being overwhelmed when the person you love is seriously ill.

In an awful and yet very consequential way, putting your needs second becomes normalized. Caregivers have many roles. You can expect that these roles and responsibilities may shift as the needs of the person you are caring for change during and after cancer treatment. It can be challenging to adapt to the changes in relationships as everyone adjusts to different priorities and new ways of being in a partnership. You may find yourself taking on tasks that your partner or family member usually performed. And it's highly likely that you may be working and/or taking care of children in addition to carrying the responsibility of caregiving the person diagnosed with cancer. You may find yourself spinning many plates in the air every day and into the night.

If the partner who's always been the one in charge, perhaps the main financial support for the family, is diagnosed with cancer, getting used to a major shift in the relationship can be difficult for both partners as it puts the dynamic of power in the spotlight. Partners who have been in charge will likely feel frustrated and helpless to maintain their usual roles, while the partners who have been put in the position of picking up the slack may find themselves feeling inadequate. There are many scenarios that get played out when a loved one gets sick, and most of them are extremely stressful. Feeling that you can communicate your fears, frustrations, and resentments becomes a key component in successfully negotiating these rough seas. It's vital that you listen to one another and remain as flexible as possible. Give yourself permission to talk openly and express your needs and be sensitive to one another's needs. When you are clear with one another, there is less possibility of misunderstanding and misinterpretation. It's a truism that people can't read our minds, and so they cannot know what you're feeling unless you tell them.

The fear of making a mistake while caring for someone is common. You feel such a deep responsibility to do the right thing that it can become paralyzing. What's true is that you are human and probably will and have made mistakes and said and done things you don't feel great about. We've all done that. It's natural, but unfortunately it's also natural to judge yourself harshly and feel like you have failed. It's important to acknowledge that you are doing the best you can and to show yourself compassion. Blaming yourself (and others) is a dead-end street when it comes to dealing with awkward and troublesome interactions or decisions. It can be a heavy burden to care for someone whose health becomes worse. You may feel like you can't ever do enough to make them better. And, sadly, you are right because no one has the power to keep someone alive. Sometimes people can feel like they have failed when someone dies. It's essential to release these thoughts and feelings and have compassion for yourself.

It's important for you to be aware of the signs that indicate you aren't really taking good care of yourself. You may notice that you feel fatigued, irritable, or depressed. Neglecting yourself won't make you feel good, so in that simple way you can help yourself by recognizing that you might need a break. Much of the advice to caregivers involves the care of the patient as well as the instructions to keep a positive attitude and handle things for the person who is dealing with cancer. While this provides a useful construct, it can also be problematic in that the needs and struggles of the caregiver continue to remain unaddressed. You may already feel overwhelmed by the demands on both your time and your energy; you don't need to add "be perfect" to your list of duties.

Be sure and give yourself credit for all that you do. It can be more familiar to spend time looking at our shortcomings and all the things we could (and should) do better. Take a moment and think about how much you give and how well you take care of things. It's important to remind yourself that you are doing the best you can and practice compassion for yourself. Stop and ask yourself, "What am I feeling and needing right now?" And then, be sure to listen . . .

> "If your compassion does not include yourself, it is incomplete."
> **—Jack Kornfield,** *Buddha's Little Instruction Book*[4]

> "Family members often cope differently and use different strategies that conflict with each other. Therapists must evaluate these differences and develop a plan to manage them that troubles the patient as little as possible. Dealing with the patient's family is not a choice, but a necessity. Relational concerns must be appraised and discussed. A surprisingly large number of patients request psychotherapy, not for their cancer, but for family and relationship concerns."
> **— Marguerite S. Lederberg and Jimmie C. Holland,** **"Supportive Psychotherapy in Cancer Care"**[5]

CAREGIVING AND CONFLICT

Dealing with cancer in troubled relationships has its own complexities. Old arguments and unresolved feelings may emerge as a relationship negotiates a cancer diagnosis. Sometimes these issues need to be brought into the light, explored, and, if possible, come to some level of resolution in order to move forward in a collaborative manner.

Under the best of circumstances, you may feel overwhelmed, burdened, and sometimes trapped while caregiving, but if you are in a troubled relationship or family, these feelings may intensify. You might feel like you got stuck with taking care of someone with whom you have conflict or someone who may not have treated you well. It can be distressing to take on the role of caregiver when you are unhappy and struggling in your relationship. You may experience both external and internal pressure to provide care, despite feeling that you don't want to do it.

It is especially important to figure out useful strategies when you become a caregiver in a conflictual relationship. It can be very helpful to find someone to share the caregiving with, or you might decide that it is in the best interests of all concerned to find another primary caregiver. From the beginning you need to clarify your limits and your boundaries in the situation and then inform people of your decisions.

We all have different communication styles—there's room for everyone. Remember that it's always helpful to express what you can and can't handle. Your perceptions are uniquely your own and being clear will help you relate in an open and respectful manner.

Pema Chödrön said, "If we learn to open our hearts, anyone, including the people who drive us crazy, can be our teacher."[6] Sometimes the toughest and most valuable lessons are learned in relationships and situations that are fraught with conflict. What Chödrön points out here is that by keeping an open heart (and mind), we are given a chance to gain a deeper understanding of ourselves and others. This isn't easy, but it may prove to be worthwhile. Perhaps by hanging in and staying as open as you can, you emerge from the obstacles you face with a newfound sense of awareness. Being able to tackle the crisis of cancer when it invades a strained relationship may be a way to bring about inner change.

Take a moment to check in with yourself about what you are thinking and feeling right now. You can incorporate this simple check-in exercise throughout your day as a way to feel connected with yourself. The workbook section at the end of this chapter will direct you in some questions about your own self-care, and it's also good to remind yourself that you have access to thinking in this way as you continue on with the book.

SHARING STORIES, FINDING COMMON GROUND

I wanted to better understand the experiences of partners, family members, and friends whose lives had been intimately touched by someone who had been diagnosed with cancer. While everyone is unique and each of us has our own way of processing our experiences, I thought I might see some universal themes. I believe that when people find common ground in the events and emotional experiences of their individual lives, it can lessen the feelings of isolation and loneliness. You may find solace and camaraderie in sharing your story with others.

I'm grateful to the people who participated in the writing of this chapter because they were open and willing to share their own stories. Some of their feelings and thoughts had never been expressed prior to answering some of the questions that I asked them. I noticed in reading over what people wrote that the word "devastated" or "devastation" appeared frequently. And yet, just as frequently, feelings of gratitude and appreciation for the relationship were expressed.

A woman who had breast cancer twice was "amazed after asking my hubby if he would answer these questions that he said yes! We just rarely talk about it, ya know? So I learned a thing or two. He is a man of few words, but at least he was willing."[7] The interaction between two people in a long-term marriage shows how "amazed" we can be at what can transpire between us when we venture beyond our usual scripts and open up a different conversation. We can create a new aliveness in our relationships when we are willing to be vulnerable with one another.

The eloquent stories of the partners, families, and friends of those with cancer speak beautifully for themselves. I include them as they were communicated to me. They contain within them the themes that bind together this group of survivors who are in distress and need to be noticed. You may find familiar words, thoughts, and feelings in the stories of these other survivors. I offer them as a way to help you feel open and comfortable with expressing your own stories.

Questions and Responses from Partners, Family Members, and Friends

Here are the questions and accompanying answers of the varied and small group of partners, friends, and family members of survivors that I interviewed for this chapter.

WHAT WAS IT LIKE WHEN YOU LEARNED YOUR PARTNER/FAMILY MEMBER/FRIEND HAD CANCER?

"Devastated."

—C. T., partner

"In hindsight, the moment was too simple, too abrupt and too wrong for the life-changing news that was about to be shared. E. called me at work from home. Her regular doctor had been vacationing out of town. E.'s allergy-like symptoms prompted an office visit to the covering doctor who then ordered an x-ray. With the results, she called to tell E. that there was a strong likelihood that the mass seen in the x-ray was lung cancer. I recall saying 'oh my God' more than I should have but mostly listening to E.'s restating what the doctor said, both of us trying to read between the lines. In her voice at that moment [was] utter disappointment, a flash of anger at having her life/our life uprooted because of some goddamn cancer[, and] the beginning of a recurring theme—frustration."

—Paul, partner

"I recall feeling total deflation, when one's physical form and brain collapse and you're nothing but a heap of skin, and a feeling of disbelief that this wasn't supposed to be happening. And I was sad thinking about what was ahead for L., the treatments, big decisions to make, and the uncertainty of it all."

—John S., partner

"It's hard to really describe just how I felt at the moment I found out Michele had cancer—shock, fear, disbelief, sadness. We had been assured by both her pediatrician and the doctor who was on call the day that we discovered a lump in her chest that they were 99% certain it wasn't cancer. The pulmonologist was just going to discuss some other diagnosis. I remember sitting there completely unconcerned for the worst as he spoke about looking at the x-rays. Michele excused herself for a moment. I looked at the doctor and simply asked what he thought it was. Then he said those words that I think most people would be devastated to hear when relating to a loved one ... she has cancer. Michele walked in almost immediately after he told me. I had about a million thoughts going

through my head. I was trying to remain composed and not look worried, which I'm sure I failed miserably at."
—**Debbie, mother**

"I was at the doctor's office with my wife when she had her biopsy. Before that, even though I was extremely worried, there was still a possibility that she didn't have cancer. Both breast surgeons were in the room when the biopsy sample was taken. My wife's doctor said that he didn't think it was malignant. When I saw the look in the other doctor's eyes, I knew the truth. I don't think I will ever forget that moment."
—**John L., partner**

"I remember it ... like being smacked in the heart with a soft piece of leather. *Smack!* Disorientation a bit. Profound immediate grief that my best friend would go through this. That I had to know *right now* how it would end, in order to prepare myself for our journey."
—**Bonnie, friend**

"On January 2, 2000, my mother was diagnosed with late stage multiple myeloma. The only words I wrote down that day were 'multiple myeloma, stem cell transplant, chemo, radiation, 1 year of treatment.' And the only thing I wondered was, 'Is my mom going to die?' I didn't ask that question that day or any of the days that followed. I knew, in that moment at the oncologist's office, that there would be some things that would be forbidden to discuss. Death would be one of them."
—**Jill, daughter**

WHAT WAS IT LIKE WHEN YOUR FAMILY MEMBER WAS IN TREATMENT FOR CANCER? HOW DID YOU FEEL?
"It was very hard to watch."
—**Debbie, mother**

"I had many concerns for quality of life during the whole process. I remember scrambling for resources for information, support groups for her, [and so forth]. It was stressful trying to support my aging parents while dealing with a complicated child who was also reacting to losing his primary babysitter and being forced suddenly into preschool."
—**Lisa, daughter**

"Concerned. There was worry about whether treatments would work, knowing there is no cure. Also worried about the toxins in the treatments and how they would affect her."
—**C. T., partner**

"I felt totally helpless. I saw the pain and suffering, even though my wife tried not to show it. I could only admire her courage and strength. Like most men, I wanted to make it better, but there was not better."
—**John L., partner**

"I helped when her partner felt 'undone' and tried to stay detached and unemotional. I visited the docs and took notes. I did not want to usurp her husband's role."
—**Susan, friend**

"Frustrating. It's inconvenient. It's cold. It takes too long. It's uncertain. It's a routine. It's a growth industry. It's a business. This is hard because you may forget what life was like before all this started. You notice how many people there for treatment arrive and leave alone."
—**Paul,** partner

"Though I knew she had lost her hair, it still came as a shock to see how small she had become, to see her in her little knit hat. That same enthusiastic smile [and] that same sparkle in her eyes was there, but behind them was a weariness. She was fighting and she was tired."
—**Wilma,** friend

"I felt overwhelmed at times—the change in routine and being mindful of all the rules and best practices for going through the treatment with the least amount of negative impact in and of itself is a lot to keep track of."
—**John S.,** partner

WHAT WAS IT LIKE WHEN YOUR LOVED ONE FINISHED TREATMENT FOR CANCER? HOW DID YOU FEEL?

"It was a challenging time, directly after treatment. Relationships and roles within the family had to be renegotiated and the growing pains associated with that were especially painful. None of us knew how to be with each other anymore. And for me, this was devastating. I assumed that whatever pathways had opened between us during treatment would continue. I was, unfortunately, wrong. In fact, after treatment we returned to not discussing anything other than on a surface level. More than the cancer and the fear of death, I think this is what was most difficult for me. I had so often heard about the transformation people can go through during cancer treatment and I witnessed that with my mom. I wasn't prepared for it to go away. I wasn't prepared for returning to a normal life to mean it would almost seem like cancer never existed. After treatment was hard because I found myself missing the mom I was beginning to get to know when she was sick and I would feel guilty for feeling that way."
—**Jill,** daughter

"Relieved but insecure as to whether it would come back."
—**C. T.,** partner

"A big relief! Time to celebrate, feel encouraged and positive. The treatment disrupts everything so completely and finishing it means everything can return to what it had previously been. Life returns to 'normal,' but it's a new normal that encompasses the disease and having gone through the treatment. The memory of it won't go away."
—**John S.,** partner

"Frustrating. It's a relief that course of treatment is over, but you know it's not really over. Everyone waits patiently for results, and you forget what life was like during treatment. You've asked about what second, third course treatments would be next. None of the answers are very thorough or helpful. Besides, maybe additional treatment won't be necessary—or advised. You hear the adjective 'palliative' for the first time."
—**Paul,** partner

"After diagnosis we had a number of very frank conversations about what we valued in each other, what we meant to each other. We basically covered any areas of conversation that needed healing, clarity, apologies, [and so forth]. Our relationship is clearer, there is more conscious respect and regard and the love, while always known to the other, has been declared more directly, openly and honestly."
—Lisa, daughter

"In some ways it was a relief. There was also the feeling that none of us knew what was next. Would the treatment, that was so devastating, work? Would the cancer come back? What would be the [long-term effects] of the treatment?"
—John L., partner

DESCRIBE YOUR FEARS AND CONCERNS.
"Her cancer experiences have affected me deeply. I have much more fear than ever before. In short, a great fear and hatred of cancer is something I now carry with me."
—Lisa, daughter

"After the diagnosis and since, I've been a lot more worried about mortality . . . my own, my kids, and my family. It was just so much to think about. How easily life could change . . . or end. It's been a couple of years, but it's hard when I have a strange pain, or my son has a cough or fever for me not to get over-the-top too paranoid. It's gotten better but it's a work in progress."
—Debbie, mother

"The first time diagnosed we had two teenagers at home, so I worried about possibly raising them alone."
—C. T., partner

"Obviously my first fear was the loss of the woman that I love. What would the treatment do to her? Would the cancer come back? Would I be able to help her the way that she needed help? My next fear was that I knew she would be different from this experience. I was concerned that we would still fit together as a couple."
—John L., partner

"I felt panic. I was scared I couldn't live without her as I was very dependent on her—she was my primary relationship."
—Susan, friend

DO YOU FEEL ANGRY?
"This [situation] has been frustrating for me and the best way for me to deal with it has been to let go."
—John S., partner

"My mother was diagnosed in December 1979. My parents were going to come out for Christmas and spend it with me. My mom was going to have surgery the day after Christmas. So, they decided to cancel the trip, and I couldn't see how postponing her surgery 1–2 days would have made any difference, and we could have spent time together as a family. The medical community didn't care. Their urgency didn't save my mother's health at all. So it made me depressed and harder on me at Christmas time. Which I still hold to this day. Thought it was always other things. Forgot about this. Writing this brought that memory back. I miss all the things we *might* have done together. As it reaches the 23rd anniversary of her death, I miss her still and again."

—Diana, daughter

"I was angry when I first heard my mom had breast cancer. I think this was a reaction to being told after the biopsy that it was not cancer. Same was true nearly five years later when she was biopsied for lung cancer. My father and I waited very anxiously in the waiting room for results and were overjoyed to learn it was not cancer. Same thing, a week later after further testing it was diagnosed as cancer. I felt angry about being told definitively that she was in the clear only to learn later what the situation really was."

—Lisa, daughter

"I have to say that I was angry, too. Angry and also fearful of my own physical and emotional vulnerability."

—John L., partner

"I also 'blamed' her. I had tried many times to warn her of dangerous behavior of birth control pills and HRT for 25 years plus. I was frustrated and also needed to find a cause to help my fear. I couldn't stand the randomness."

—Susan, friend

DO YOU STILL WORRY?
"Yes."

—C. T., partner

"I try not to, but it's impossible not to think about it. Whenever my wife goes in for a check-up or mammogram, I think about the negative possibilities."

—John L., partner

"I believe, without one doubt, that my mom could survive cancer again. I don't think my dad could. I worry a lot about him. The two rounds of cancer almost killed him, I shudder to think what a third would do."

—Jill, daughter

"I worry for her but even more I worry for myself, I'm not proud to say. I don't feel as safe since her diagnosis. I feel almost immobilized about how to proceed with genetic testing so I have chosen to do nothing but monthly breast exams and yearly mammograms."

—Lisa, daughter

"About what? I may get cancer or not! If asked, I would not get the cancer marker test done. I don't want to know—what, so I can watch myself die and worry, instead of living my life?"

—Diana, daughter

"I worry sometimes, but it's not an acute kind of worry that surfaces every day. Cancer is everywhere, and for me, there's no way to live a balanced, worry-free life without putting cancer in a compartment in my mind."
—**John S.,** partner

"It may not be worry, but most times I drive past each of the three hospitals where treatments or surgeries were performed, I think about the stream of people with cancer that have come and gone, some brilliant physicians who I credit with extending E.'s life for over three years during which good life was lived and lots of friends and relatives stumbled through the experience, some with such humanity and grace, others as best they could."
—**Paul,** partner

HOW HAS YOUR RELATIONSHIP CHANGED SINCE THE CANCER DIAGNOSIS?

"On good days, I feel guilty for being free to have fun while he's feeling down, and on bad days, I feel overwhelmed by sadness and fear on my brother's behalf. . . . Sharing these thoughts with him now feels selfish."
—**Ryan Rose Weaver, "What Should Siblings Do in the Face of Cancer?"**[8]

"I think our relationship is stronger in many ways. I certainly don't take it for granted. I do still find that we are adjusting to the current reality of cancer survivorship."
—**John L.,** partner

"My relationship with my mother post-cancer is evolving. The closet I ever felt to her remains during the time of her treatment. It has been a difficult road for our relationship in the years that have followed. The birth of my daughter has helped to heal that though. She says 'I love you,' the whole family says 'I love you' now, so I take this as a gift from cancer."
—**Jill,** daughter

"It was certainly an intimate and intense shared experience and going through it together made us closer. Having gotten through something as horrible as a cancer diagnosis and the treatment, with the physical and emotional exhaustion that weaves in and out of it, we can get through anything."
—**John S.,** partner

"It has changed some because of her other physical limitations and her not being as mobile as she used to be so that the times between 1-to-1 visits has increased because I seem to be busier that I was in years past. Honestly, most of the time I am sad to admit, I forget she went through cancer. Makes me realize in this moment that I need to check in with her about that."
—**Sandra,** friend

"E. died late in the morning on Friday, November 18th, 2005. Stripped to the essentials and wonder of being alive, an already good relationship got better. We spent 38 consecutive months being more in the moment that most couples do in a lifetime."
—**Paul,** partner

"Cheryl's cancer, while it has brought up fears about losing her, has reminded me that loving fiercely is what my heart really wants to do. If it breaks again, so be it. Missing out on this precious friendship as a way to avoid pain would be its own form of heartbreak and feel much worse. Her cancer added to the realness of our relationship."
—Wilma, friend

"I worry more about her health."
—C. T., partner

"After treatment, I got more independent. I didn't need her as much; not as needy. She became a dear friend, not a life support."
—Susan, friend

"I'm aware that death is more present than not in our lives now, that I feel like some part of us is more conscious of the more intense place we go to."
—Bonnie, friend

WHAT HAS IT BEEN LIKE SINCE THEY FINISHED TREATMENT?

"Although every day my heart felt like it was rebreaking into a thousand pieces watching her suffering, I was grateful that I had a job. I had a purpose for being there with her and I liked that I could do something to help, in whatever small way that was. I'm proud of her desire to live and her fight."
—Jill, daughter

"I've experienced a lot of death in my life, it seems. I'm to the point that the death of someone I love feels like a well-worn road with too many familiar potholes and winding turns."
—Wilma, friend

"Few experiences are as powerful as cancer to learn so much—both good and otherwise—about one's friends. What came up for me? I was always faithful, always present. I felt trusted."
—Paul, partner

"Cheryl reminded me that this *was* about me, about my best friend and me. I've had a series of cancer and AIDS deaths in the past ten years and Cheryl was aware of that with me. I don't know what she didn't tell me, if anything, about her experience, illness, prognosis, [and so on], but my bet is that I got it all. I hope so."
—Bonnie, friend

"Overall, knowing so many women going through breast cancer around the same time was shocking and gave me pause. I thought about the fact that all the people in my Mom's generation in our family had died of cancer and how I could have been and still could be one of them. Just having people close to me get breast cancer made it more of a reality and the closeness of the friendships intensified the feelings. Currently I find myself in awe of how my friends have handled their recovery and wonder if I could be that strong, open, and honest. Being in conversations about serious stuff and possible death increases the intimacy of the relationship and that is certainly something I experienced in every case.

A deeper knowing of the person and their strengths and vulnerabilities changed things in important ways."
—Sandra, friend

"Other than my fear of loss, I was faced, yet again, with my own mortality."
—John L., partner

You've heard feelings of fear, anger, love, worry, and guilt expressed on these pages. Do you find that there were some responses that touched you? What sorts of thoughts and feelings are emerging for you as you read their stories?

In some of the stories that were shared here, anger seemed to compensate for deep feelings of helplessness. Anger and frustration with the medical system and the types of treatment showed up in people's comments. The experience of uncertainty created anguish as these people stood by and watched the situation unfold. And for those of you in difficult relationships, the anger and frustration can be especially draining and toxic.

The ideal of the perfect and loving caregiving relationship can be oppressive. This version of tyranny involves the pressure of being good and loving at all costs. At times self-sacrifice may be elevated to distinctly unhealthy levels, causing the caregiver to fall ill from exhaustion. Expressing that caregiving can feel obligatory and may create the experience of feeling trapped is difficult to share.

Fear arises continually throughout the stories expressed by partners, friends, and family members: fear of loss, fear of change, fear of mortality. It's common for others to become anxious over their own health, concerned about their own issues of mortality and dealing with their own struggles with uncertainty. All of the people who participated indicated that being close to someone with cancer touches your emotional life in deep and impactful ways.

Many of the people who contributed their stories felt pride in watching the patients fight for their lives. They felt inspired and sometimes moved to make changes in their own lives based on witnessing the courage of the person who they cared for. And once that fight was over, some of the same feelings of uncertainty arose. Treatment is over, now what? Now we wait . . .

But you don't really want to just sit and wait, you want to get on with your life. Cancer often affects, and at times can change, future hopes, dreams, and plans that people share. Old stories of what we believed would happen can change. However, that does not necessarily mean that new hopes, dreams, and plans cannot become the new stories you create in your relationships.

> "If only healing after cancer caregiving were as fast and predictable as recovering from a scratch or a bruise. After caregiving ends, you'll find yourself grieving, regardless of whether your care recipient has died, fears potential recurrence, or has been declared cancer free."
> **—Deborah J. Cornwall, "How Cancer Caregivers Heals"[9]**

> "I have woven a parachute out of everything broken."
> **—William Stafford, "Any Time"[10]**

WORKBOOK SECTION: TELL YOUR STORY
FOR PARTNERS, FAMILY MEMBERS, AND FRIENDS

> "From caring comes courage."
> **—Lao Tzu**

After the person you care for has finished treatment for cancer, many of you may still feel unfinished with what has just happened for you. Indeed, you may not have had a chance to understand your own experience, let alone have had the time or energy to express it to anyone else. It's likely that you feel a need to connect with yourself to find out where you are now in your life. After allowing yourself to discover your own story, you may find yourself more able to speak about your experiences so that you can better understand and begin to integrate them into your life as you move forward.

The following questions are designed to help you reflect on your experience and the significant impact of cancer in your life. There aren't any right or wrong answers. I invite you to use this workbook as a way to give yourself a place for needed reflection. Your self-care is essential and the opportunity for you to contemplate and identify the ways that you can care for yourself is provided in this section. Please give yourself time and space to be with these narrative questions. And if you feel it would be helpful, share what you discover with your partner, families, and friends. By expressing your own story, you can feel more connected with yourself and with others.

The workbook is divided into separate sections for partners, family members, young children, and friends, as there are different needs in each type of relationship.

TELL YOUR STORY FOR PARTNERS

1.   How are you doing?

2.   What was it like when you first learned that your partner was diagnosed
     with cancer?

3. How do you support yourself? Do you find it hard to focus on your own needs and wants?

4. What has it been like for you to have your partner diagnosed with cancer?

5. What feelings and issues arose for you?

6. Describe your fears and concerns.

7. What was it like for you when your partner was in treatment?

8. What has it been like since your partner finished treatment?

9. What is it like if you are someone whose partner is living with cancer?

10. What do you feel worried and afraid about?

11. How has your relationship with your partner changed since the cancer diagnosis?

12. Are there issues or concerns that you have about intimacy in your relationship? Do you feel comfortable talking with your partner about sexuality?

13. Have there been issues around fertility that have affected your relationship? If so, how has this impacted you?

14. Do you feel pressured to always be strong and supportive?

15. Do you ever feel resentful or guilty? What is that like for you?

16. What do you feel about your quality of life?

17. Do you feel that you have a place to talk openly about your concerns? How do you identify and find the resources your need?

18. How are things for you now?

19. How do you and your partner look at future plans?

20. Do you have ways you take care of yourself? What are they? Make a list so that you have a reference that you can rely on to help you support yourself. This list can be revisited whenever you feel the need to make changes in how you take care of yourself.

TELL YOUR STORY FOR FAMILY MEMBERS

1.   How are you?

2.   What was it like for you when your family member was diagnosed with cancer?

3. How do you feel your family was affected by someone who was going through treatment for cancer?

4. How has it been for you and your family since your family member finished treatment?

5. Are you in a family with someone who is living with cancer? How does that impact you?

6. Are you a parent of a cancer survivor? How are you doing? Are you finding the support that you need in dealing with the life-threatening illness of your child or young adult?

7. Do you find it difficult to focus on your own needs and wants?

8. What feelings and issues are present for you?

9.   What are your fears and concerns?

10. Do you still worry?

11. Do you ever feel resentful or guilty? What is that like for you?

12. Do you feel that you get the support you need to help you deal with these issues? How do you identify and find the resources you need?

13. Are you in the role of a caregiver? If so, what is that like for you?

14. Do you have ways you take care of yourself? What are they? Make a list so that you have a reference that you can rely on to help you support yourself. This list can be revisited whenever you feel the need to make changes in how you take care of yourself.

TELL YOUR STORY FOR YOUNG CHILDREN OF CANCER SURVIVORS

This workbook section is designed for a parent or other family member, medical practitioner, psychotherapist or social worker, or other adult to give to a young child of someone who has survived or lives with cancer. This may be given as an interview or, if the child is old enough, be given as a handout for the child to fill out and bring back to share. Art materials, toys, sand tray, or other nonwritten tools may be helpful. It is especially important to allow children to access their thoughts and feelings in a nonlinear fashion. In truth, little ones live more in the world of story and play, so it is a natural way for them to communicate. As adults, we can all learn from the ways in which children express themselves.

1. How are you?

2. Tell me a story about your family. Would you like to draw a picture of your family?

3. Do you sometimes feel scared? Can you tell me about that or would you like to show me or draw a picture?

4. Tell me about a really good day when you had a lot of fun. What was the best part of that day?

5. Tell me about a really bad day when you didn't feel very good. What was the worst part of that day?

6. Do you sleep well? Do you sometimes have bad dreams? Can you tell me about them or show me or draw a bad dream?

7. Do you ever feel worried or does your tummy hurt sometimes for no reason?

8. If you could have any wish, what would you wish for?

9. If you could have any superpower, what would you pick?

10. If we could take an airplane and go on an adventure to anywhere, where would we go?

SURVIVING THE STORM

1. Describe the moment when you learned that your friend had cancer.

2. What was the relationship like when your friend had cancer?

3. What was the relationship like after your friend finished treatment?

4. Do you have friend who is living with cancer? What is that like for you?

5. How has your relationship changed?

6. Do you sometimes struggle with feelings about your friend being unavailable because he or she is ill? What's that like for you?

7. What feelings and issues arose for you?

8. Do you still worry?

9. Do you ever feel resentful or guilty? What is that like for you?

10. Can you talk openly with your friend about these feelings? Are you concerned about saying the right or wrong thing?

11. If you could say anything to your friend about your experience, what would you say? Let yourself be as uncensored as possible. You can decide whether you want to share this with your friend after you have given yourself the chance to express yourself.

NOTES

1. Ronald Wallace, "The Truth," in *Long for This World: New and Selected Poems* (Pittsburgh, PA: University of Pittsburg Press, 2003), 98. Used by permission of the University of Pittsburg Press. © 2003 by Ronald Wallace.

2. American Society of Clinical Oncology (ASCO), "Post-Traumatic Stress Disorder and Cancer," Cancer.net, January 2016, www.cancer.net/survivorship/life-after-cancer/post-traumatic-stress-disorder-and-cancer.

3. Chief Seattle, BrainyQuote.com, Xplore Inc, 2016, www.brainyquote.com/quotes/authors/c/chief_seattle.html, accessed October 26, 2016. "Seattle" was a Native American Suquamish tribal chief.

4. Jack Kornfield, *Buddha's Little Instruction Book* (New York: Bantam, 1994), 28. Used by permission of Bantam Books, an imprint of Random House, a division of Penguin Random House, LLC. All rights reserved. Any third party use of this material, outside this publication, is prohibited. Interested parties must apply to Penguin Random House LLC for permission. © 1994 by Jack Kornfield.

5. Marguerite S. Lederberg and Jimmie C. Holland, "Supportive Psychotherapy in Cancer Care: An Essential Ingredient of All Therapy," in *Handbook of Psychotherapy in Cancer Care*, ed. Maggie Watson and David W. Kissane (Chichester, UK: Wiley-Blackwell, 2011), 1–14. Used by permission of John Wiley & Sons, a member of the Perseus Books Group. © 2011 by John Wiley & Sons, Ltd.

6. Pema Chödrön, *When Things Fall Apart: Heart Advice for Difficult Times* (Boulder, CO: Shambhala, 1997), 65-66. Used by permission of The Permissions Company, Inc. on behalf of Shambhala Publications Inc., Boulder, Colorado, www.shambhala.com. © 1997 by Pema Chödrön.

7. Personal interview with author.

8. Ryan Rose Weaver, "What Should Siblings Do in the Face of Cancer?" Roswell Park Cancer Institute (blog), February 22, 2013, www.roswellpark.org/cancertalk/201302/what-should-siblings-do-face-cancer.

9. Deborah J. Cornwall, "How Cancer Caregivers Heal," Cancer Knowledge Network, August 1, 2013, https://cancerkn.com/how-cancer-caregivers-heal/.

10. William Stafford, "Any Time" in *The Way It Is: New & Selected Poems* (Minneapolis, MN: Graywolf Press, 1998), 127. Used by permission of The Permissions Company, Inc., on behalf of Graywolf Press, Minneapolis, Minnesota, www.graywolfpress.org. © 1970, 1998 by William Stafford and the Estate of William Stafford.

PLEASE LISTEN! HOW TO TALK WITH YOUR HEALTHCARE TEAM

7

I am not this hair,
I am not this skin,
I am the soul that lives within.
—Rumi

ONCE UPON A TIME, A THREE-YEAR-OLD GIRL received a toy stethoscope and decided to perform a health examination on her mother, who was living with stage IV colon cancer. She knew that her mother was very sick and wanted to care for her by offering her help. Without asking her mother (the patient) any questions or taking the time to listen to her story, the little girl (the doctor) began her exam. Following a very serious and silent going over, checking her mother by physically thumping her body and then listening through her stethoscope, the child declared that she had reached a diagnosis. Without another word, she turned her back on her patient (her mother) and ran to her toy computer to begin madly entering her findings into the database in the computerized healthcare record system.

This true story reminds us that the relationship between provider and patient is key to holistic healing. Relationships are healing when people acknowledge one another as human beings who accept and respect one another. And yet all too often, feeling seen and heard by your healthcare team can be a challenging experience. There is rarely time for you to tell your provider your story and show them who you are as a person, not just an illness. Even just getting a chance to spend enough time discussing what is currently happening is not something that occurs frequently. While I have tremendous empathy for the heavy load of the clinicians in the oncology world, you, the patient, deserve to be treated and respected as a human being who is dealing with very real life and death concerns. In this chapter, we'll look at some of the ways in which you can take charge of your healthcare and also feel more connected with those who are providing your care.

We all want our concerns to be met with understanding and compassion. Being able to get the information you need about your health is a human right. When you feel valued as a person and are treated with respect, you feel well cared for by your provider. While some of us may want a more relational style with our providers and others simply want them to be technicians and get the job done quickly (and successfully), we all share a desire for clear communication. Communication is very personal and at its best, it doesn't feel canned, dogmatic, or condescending. Trusting your own needs and wants, as well as honoring the communication style that best suites you, helps you to choose not only the providers who work for you, but with you.

Warfield Theobald Longcope, physician-in-chief of Johns Hopkins Hospital from 1922 to 1946, once said, "Each patient ought to feel somewhat the better after the physician's visit, irrespective of the nature of the illness."[1] This chapter will explore the ways in which you can feel more effective in your communication with your healthcare team. Remember that you do have permission to ask questions, request what you need, and get the kind of care you deserve.

DON'T BE AFRAID TO SPEAK UP!

How do I become my own expert? How can I learn to be my own advocate? When do I let my healthcare team make the decisions and when do I question the course of action that is being taken? These are questions you've probably asked yourself and others. Communicating with your healthcare team can be a daunting task. Getting caught in voicemail hell or not getting a response in the aftermath of having sent numerous emails is an all too familiar experience.

Don't be afraid to speak up. It's important for you to let your doctor know if you don't understand something. Remember that there are no stupid questions and that it's okay to ask for clarification. Sometimes medical terms are used that none of us understand, and it's okay to ask your provider to speak in a language that you can understand.

Tell your provider when you feel you need more time to talk about what is going on for you. By doing this ahead of time, you may be able to speak with one of his or her assistants or with a nurse. If this doesn't work, schedule another appointment. What's important is that you don't give up on what you need. By asking for more time with your provider, you can offer him or her the narrative you have created in the workbook sections of this book; you are telling your provider *your* story. This helps your doctor know and understand you as a complete person, not just a cancer patient.

> "It is better to let someone walk away from you than all over you."
> **—Anonymous**

Another way to help yourself feel more in charge is to bring someone with you to your appointments. It can be difficult to be completely present if you're feeling anxious about meeting with your provider. And when you can't be as fully present as possible, you miss information that is important for you to understand. It can be very helpful to bring someone along with you who can take notes, ask questions about things you may not remember to ask, and fill in information that you may not think of in the moment. It also helps you to be more engaged in the conversation if another person is writing down both the questions and the responses or, prior to your visit, you may also ask if it's alright to record the appointment. Having another person in the room with you can give you the feeling of someone "being in your corner" and for many of us that gives us the support and encouragement we need to voice our concerns.

TAKING RESPONSIBILITY FOR YOUR PART

I was at a first appointment for an evaluation of some tests for some back problems I was dealing with. While the physician's assistant was pleasant, he was a bit like the little girl at the beginning of this chapter and spent quite of bit of time at the computer terminal rather than interacting with me. After he examined my reports, he asked me if I would prefer a male or female physician referral.

"I would like someone who is human," I told him, "and that can be a person who is either male or female." The man's demeanor immediately switched, and he gave me a rather large grin. From that moment on, we began a completely different interaction, which was vulnerable, humorous, and personal. We actually talked about his life as well as mine. When he needed to make notes on his computer, he apologized for turning away.

Ask to be treated like a human being and treat your provider with that same respect and care. This is your responsibility in your relationship with your provider. It may not always end as warmly and successfully as my experience did, but it's worth taking a chance. Ask for what you need and then be sure to listen to your provider's responses. If you don't understand something, ask for clarification. Remember, there are no stupid questions, and it's vital that you understand what is happening in order for you to be an advocate for your own care. Don't be dissuaded by impatience or accept that there is a lack of time to fully respond to you.

Sometimes it can be useful to let your provider ask questions first. Providers are usually somewhat bound to a checklist of standard questions of things that they need to document, so it can be expedient to follow along with protocol. However, you don't need to be passive in this process. If something isn't right or doesn't really fit with your own situation, let the provider know. Question their questions and ask your own if the interview isn't feeling relevant to your issues. Give yourself the authority to represent your body and your life in the ways that work for you.

If you get cut off during the interview, insist that your concerns and questions be heard. However, recognize when you may be asking for answers that simply aren't there for the provider to give. Medicine is not an exact science, and providers deal with uncertainty just like you do. You can't expect your provider to wave a wand of certainty over an uncertain outcome. Keep in mind that your physician is a human being who is invested in helping you in your healing process. These people have dedicated their lives to helping others and carry a tremendous amount of responsibility. By relating to them in a compassionate manner, you play your part in creating a healing relationship. An empathic stance helps to open a conversation that builds a respectful relationship and brings about rewarding resolutions.

> "Be who you are, say what you feel because those who mind don't matter and those who matter don't mind."
> **—Anonymous**

DR. GOOGLE AND SCANXIETY

You've finished your treatment for cancer and it's time to move back out into a world that is no longer filled with the structure of frequent appointments or a treatment schedule that has become a familiar way of life. You've been declared in remission, and your contact with your oncology team will decrease. In some cases, you may only have yearly visits. But it's more likely that you've now entered a period of monitoring your health with follow-up visits, which often include blood tests, physical checkups, scans, and other evaluative tools and examinations. This can be the moment I mentioned earlier in the book where you feel like you have fallen off a cliff without being tethered to the climbing ropes of the healthcare team members who have held you throughout your treatment. This is when many of us turn to Dr. Google.

Turning to the Internet is a common response to the lack of control you feel after you have been following a clear plan of action that is no longer in place. We start consulting Internet sites to fill in the questions and concerns that arise when our healthcare team isn't as nearby as before and watching us as closely, and without this, we fear that anything could happen. Our thoughts roil around in our heads: "Cancer unexpectedly happened before, it could happen again." You may even begin making appointments with Dr. Google.

Dr. Google can be found in many places online and can be either helpful or traumatizing, depending upon the accuracy and quality of information you research. As with anything on the Web, there are valid and valuable sources, as well as those whose information is sketchy at best and terrifyingly catastrophic at worst. Prior to engaging in this type of online activity, you may want to ask your provider about valid Internet sites or resources that deal with your type of cancer. I also include resources at the back of this book to help you navigate these sites. While information is a key to self-advocacy, discernment is also critical to any Internet search. Present any questions that might come up as a way for you to educate yourself, not as a challenge to your provider's knowledge. This will make any conversation about your findings a path to deeper understanding between you and your provider and not an argument about who knows best.

Scanxiety is anxiety suffered while waiting for the results of an important medical scan, and it can also apply to other diagnostic tests. The anxiety of living with uncertainty is triggered during these waiting periods. As a survivor, you have negative associations with these tests, and it can be triggering to wait, once again, for results. Again, in these instances, it's tempting to run right to the Internet for answers, either when we have received a diagnosis or are experiencing symptoms that we don't understand. This is an understandable reaction to the uncertainty of living in the post-treatment world. But do exercise caution. Notice when your thoughts begin to run wild and you tell yourself scary stories that only make you more anxious and apprehensive. Turn off the horror show on your computer screen and take a breath. Anxiety and worry are not soothed by obsessively seeking information and viewing images that frighten you. Take care of your anxiety by staying in touch with how you are feeling and reacting and make adjustments by paying attention to your level of distress.

Name your anxiety, recognize it as an emotional state like any other, and remind yourself that you can make choices about how much power you hand over to it. You are human, you've had cancer, you get anxious, and that's normal. Sometimes expressing your fears out loud releases them so that you aren't carrying all that anxiety inside yourself. Give yourself permission to talk with people whom you trust to listen to your fears. It's a good idea to surround yourself with people who are comfortable with your feelings, can listen to you, help reassure you, and put you at ease. You also have the option to talk with a professional of your choice who can listen and assist you in finding your own ways to deal with your anxieties, one who accepts that anxiety is a normal reaction for you to experience. A word of caution here, too: I have listened to far too many stories in which people have been patronized for their anxiety and treated like they were abnormal or crazy. I know of one woman who was even offered an antipsychotic medication when she spoke with her provider about her feelings of anxiety. Thankfully, she didn't take it. She was able to talk about her concerns and work in other ways to care for herself. So trust yourself in these instances too. If you speak to a provider who's not empathic or who makes you feel crazy, see if you can find someone else to connect to.

THINK OUTSIDE THE BOX

You're probably familiar with the distress screening checklists that are generally used to assess how you are doing when you've finished cancer treatment. Helpful, yes, but the small boxes aren't big enough to contain and express your personal experience. You can't tell a story within a small box. You don't have to remain within the confines of these limited structures. Give yourself the choice to color outside the lines and reveal yourself as a human being, not just a cancer patient.

Part of revealing yourself involves advocating for yourself so that you have a stake in your own treatment. When I asked a group of breast cancer survivors on Facebook what had worked for them when it came to communicating with their providers, one woman said, "interpretive dance." I found this tongue-in-cheek response not only hilarious, but right on target. How well your providers know you depends on how well you introduce yourself to them. While getting to know them doesn't guarantee that you will be seen as the whole person you are, it's certainly gives you a better chance to advocate for yourself. Don't let yourself become a number. The more you let yourself be known, the more present you are, and the more in charge you will feel. Developing a strong sense of your own inner presence allows you the spaciousness and clarity to show up for yourself and feel empowered.

WORKBOOK SECTION: HOW TO COMMUNICATE WITH YOUR HEALTHCARE TEAMS

Telling Your Story: Create Your Own Survivor Care Plan

Although it is a requirement for accredited cancer providers to see that every cancer survivor receives a survivor care plan, it doesn't always happen. This workbook section can help you organize your health information, such as dates, diagnosis, treatment issues, and questions, and also give you a narrative record of your experiences, which can serve as your own survivor care plan. Cancer survivorship is (hopefully) a long-term process, and the following workbook section can be used over the months and years of post-treatment for clarification and personal expression. It's helpful to refer to the workbook sections in this book for use any time you are having an in-depth or personal conversation with your provider.

Use the questions in this section as a guideline to help you prepare for your appointments, as well as help formulate your thoughts on what you need with and from your provider. Having a structure can assist you in forming satisfying relationships with your providers.

"The Essentials" listed in the following section can serve as a logistical and pragmatic checklist. These are things to remember or do for each appointment. The next set of questions presented are designed to help you negotiate the initial stages of diagnosis and treatment and to help you gain information, not only about your treatments but ways to interview your provider to see if he or she is a match for you. The third set of questions relates to what to expect in post-treatment, as well as what you might want and need for yourself in that phase of a cancer diagnosis. If you want to keep this information in a central place, make notes in this workbook and update it periodically. If you prefer, you can bring a separate notebook or use your phone to record the information. Whatever you choose, you might find it helpful to keep your information in a single document to make it easy and accessible.

The Essentials: What to Remember for Every Medical Appointment

☐ Bring your insurance card and ID to your appointment.

☐ Be prepared to talk about any changes in your health, new test results, or new symptoms.

☐ Bring a list of your medications (you can also take photos on your phone). Be sure to tell your doctor about any negative reactions you have had to medications or other treatments.

☐ Bring your calendar so that you can schedule other appointments. This helps save time and the frustration of trying to make appointments via telephone or email.

Questions to Ask Your Doctor

The initial entry into cancer treatment is both confusing and daunting. It's hard to even know what to ask, let alone to have any idea of what you need. Having some kind of simple structure to begin with can help you find your way through this bewildering time. Here are some questions to ask your doctor, physician's assistant, or nurse to help you understand your treatment and follow-up care:

• What is my specific diagnosis?

• Have you treated other patients with my type of cancer?

- What are my treatment options?

- What is the recommended treatment?

- How often will I receive treatment? Where will I go for my treatments? How long will my treatments take?

- What are the possible side effects?

- What are the possible benefits and risks of this treatment?

- If I have questions during my treatment and my doctor is not available, who can I ask? Who can I call? For example, if you are not available, is a nurse, social worker, or other specialist available? (Get the phone number including extension and record it here for easy reference.)

- Is there any information that I can read about this treatment or procedure? (This is how you can ask about valid resources both on and off the Internet.)

- How do you feel about integrative treatments, such as acupuncture? (It is important to tell your provider that you use these types of integrative practices in order to coordinate different types of care. By asking this question you can find out up front if your doctor is open to working with integrative treatments.)

- Is there anything else I should know? (You can also use some time to tell your providers what you feel is useful for them to know. You may want to make some notes here prior to your appointment or refer to your Tell Your Story workbook section.)

Questions about Post-Treatment: What Happens as I Move On?

There is very little available information for post-treatment concerns, and some facilities have little or nothing at all to offer people as they move into the survivor phase of a cancer diagnosis. Yet follow-up care is necessary because you will need to pay careful attention to your health for the remainder of your life. The main purpose for medical follow-up care is to check for recurrence or metastasis. Follow-up care visits are also important to help in the prevention or early detection of other types of cancer. These appointments address any collateral damage you have that is caused by cancer or its treatment, and to check for other physical effects that may appear after the end of your treatment. These might include things such as chemotherapy-induced peripheral neuropathy, lymphedema, heart issues, and weight gain or loss.

There should also be a thorough focus on the social and emotional concerns you may have or develop as you move further away from your cancer treatment. This area of concern is more complex than the standard medical record and less linear in nature. Therefore, it demands an approach that includes both open-ended questions and room for a narrative structure that includes personal information. You can ask to be given a referral to a psychotherapist, social worker, or cancer survivor group as an alternative for you to find the help you need.

Questions to ask your provider as you enter the post-treatment phase of cancer:

• How often should I have follow-up appointments? What kinds of tests will I have? Tell me about the post-treatment care you think I will need.

- Who should I see for my follow-up cancer care?

- What symptoms should I watch for?

- How can I tell if symptoms such as pain, fatigue, or any other physical difficulties are something to be concerned about? What should I pay attention to?

- Should I be concerned about difficulties with memory and concentration?

- If I develop any symptoms, who should I call?

- What are the chances that my cancer will come back, or that I will get another type of cancer?

- What are the common long-term and late effects of the treatment I received?

- How do you suggest that I explore the emotional impact of my cancer experience? Do you have referrals for this kind of help?

These questions can help you focus and will give you a structure for thinking about your needs and wants as you move into post-treatment. As you read this book and explore your experience in the workbook sections, you may develop your own list of questions and concerns. You can use the space that follows to write those down and refer to them when you are talking with your healthcare team.

Questions, Thoughts, Ideas, and Feelings: My Concerns

In the end, you are your own expert when it comes to how well you know your body, your mind, and yourself. The most effective way to advocate for yourself is to bring your own self-awareness to your conversations with your healthcare providers. You co-create a healing relationship when there is collaboration between the expertise and knowledge of your provider and your own expert opinion of your personal experience.

> "You need a good bedside manner with doctors or you will get nowhere."
> —**William S. Burroughs**, *Junky*[2]

NOTES

1. "Warfield Theobald Longcope," in *The Oxford Dictionary of Medical Quotations*, ed. Peter McDonald (Oxford, UK: Oxford University Press, 2004), 61.
2. William S. Burroughs, *Junky* (New York: Grove Press, 2003), 26. Used by permission of Grove/Atlantic, Inc. Any third party use of this material, outside this publication, is prohibited. © 1953 by A.A. Wyn, Inc.; 1977, 1981 by William S. Burroughs; 2003 by the Estate of William S. Burroughs.

PINK HAS A SHADOW

DARK HUMOR, BAD LINES, AND CANCER

If you have your health, you have everything
is something that's said to cheer you up
when you come home and find your lover
arched over a stranger in a scarlet thong.
Or it could be you lose your job at Happy Nails
because you can't stop smudging the stars
on those ten teeny American flags.
I don't begrudge you your extravagant vitality.
May it blossom like a cherry tree. May the petals
of your cardiovascular excellence
and the accordion polka of your lungs
sweeten the mornings of your loneliness.
But for the ill, for you with nerves that fire
like a rusted-out burner on an old barbecue,
with bones as brittle as spun sugar,
with a migraine hammering like a blacksmith
in the flaming forge of your skull,
may you be spared from friends who say,
God doesn't give you more than you can handle
and ask what gifts being sick has brought you.
May they just keep their mouths shut
and give you French chocolates and daffodils
and maybe a small, original Matisse,
say, Open Window, Collioure, *so you can look out*
at the boats floating on the dappled pink water.
—Ellen Bass, "French Chocolates"[1]

I REMEMBER HEARING ABOUT "THE GIFT OF CANCER" before I had cancer. Being a person who believes in transformation, I thought it had a certain ethereal elegance to it. I mean, look at Lance Armstrong. I thought (before the confessions of all that steroid use), "He won the Tour de France and started a foundation." Other famous people had come forward with messages of profound learning leading to life changes. Their stories were often deeply moving. They spoke of misery and affliction, which had not been chosen but rather thrust upon them. The courage of their choices in the face of trauma and suffering was inspirational. Yes, cancer was a life-threatening disease, and yet it appeared to be a precious present wrapped in a cloak of darkness for so many!

When I was told I had an aggressive breast cancer, my first thought was not, "Thank you, I am absolutely thrilled with this gift!" It was all I could do not to hyperventilate, keel over, and hit my head. I called my husband. He was not excited either. We did not open a bottle of champagne and dance wildly about the room in elation. Nor were we happy about having to tell our then fourteen-year-old son the news. As an ordinary woman living an ordinary life, I just kept putting one foot in front of the other, hoping that my ordinary life, which suddenly seemed remarkably precious, would continue.

For me and anyone with a new cancer diagnosis, you start wondering the moment after diagnosis if you are going to die from this disease. The thoughts and feelings that follow circle around what it will be like to go through cancer treatment. You enter a basic mode of survival with little internal bandwidth for considering the gifts that may come from this life-changing event. Fairly soon after diagnosis, I began a serious and debilitating course of treatment that I hoped would end as an exchange for "the gift of remission." I am grateful that ultimately I did receive this gift and all that it has taught me, but even now I still would have rather skipped the cancer.

Much has been written, talked about, filmed, photographed, described, and blogged chronicling the transformative experience of cancer. Without question, heroic memoirs and miracles do inspire us to trudge on through the muck of illness. You often read about cancer survivors flipping their lives into something more meaningful than they had ever dreamed possible. But we'll leave those stories to another page.

How does your life change after cancer? Even more evocatively, how are *you* changed after cancer?

After I lost my long, fine, corkscrew curls, my hair came back short, and with the help of a bit of product, spiky. Those who hadn't seen me for a while didn't recognize me. If I knew them at all, I would explain that I had lost my hair during cancer treatment. If I didn't know them, well, I merely said, "Yes, I look a bit different." Complete strangers continue to stop me on the street or in the store to tell me how much they love my hair and asking, "Who does it?" I tell them, "This is a chemo cut, the most expensive haircut I ever got." Glassy-eyed, they often back away from me probably thinking, "Don't want to go to that salon!"

Looking different on the outside wasn't my only change. I was no stranger to sitting with mortality, my own and that of others. Considering my age—fifty-five—my own mortality was really still a concept, not something I felt I'd be facing so soon. But for me, and for anyone receiving a life-threatening diagnosis, whatever intellectual concept of death we've held suddenly flies out of the window when we are smacked with the reality of facing our mortality head on. It's a bit unnerving, to say the least. People make comments such as, "we're all going to die," which imply that it's really no big deal, that we're all doomed anyway, so stop complaining. Yes, we're all going to die, but it's a bit different when you draw the short straw of cancer. While I really, really wanted to become a better person, I sometimes felt pressured by the expectation (my own and those of others) of some profound transformation. I knew there was an opportunity for immense personal growth, but it's complicated by the threat of death that might cut short whatever plans we make.

There are entire books and blogs devoted to what to say and what not to say when someone has cancer. Apparently no one is reading them because the reports of well-meaning and awkward remarks just keep on coming. One of my favorite lines comes from John Green's book *The Fault in Our Stars*: " 'I don't think you're dying,' I said. 'I think you've just got a touch of cancer.' "[2]

Several times I had conversations starting with: "Oh, it's just breast cancer . . . at least it's not in your liver . . . it could be worse, you have the good cancer." Once again I felt a tad guilty that I was not making the most of my cancer gift. It was extremely tempting to not snap back with, "Wow, I hadn't thought of that, I sure feel better now. I never knew until I had breast cancer that it was the good one to get."

It's not unusual to be told, "I know exactly how you feel." This is nearly always followed by numerous stories of friends, family members, cousin-of-the-person-at-the-market, daughter-of-my-mechanic's-roommate's-sister who supposedly have or had the same cancer you do and who are still around after fifteen years. Occasionally a dourer tale is told of my brother's-boss's-wife's-best friend who died a terrible death. My all-time favorite is, "I understand what you're going through, my dog had cancer."

But it's not only the people diagnosed with cancer who struggle with knowing what to say and what not to say. There are cancer patients who are unable to talk about the seriousness of what is happening for them, including fears of leaving their partners, families, and others. People may feel caught in a code of silence that can feel disorienting and sometimes a bit crazy. This strained and frustrating lack of communication dispels the myth of the perfect, loving family clasping hands and sharing feelings with one another. A comment from the daughter of a cancer patient, Jill, illustrates this perfectly: "Comforting my mother seemed unnatural. I couldn't expect comfort from her. So, regrettably I didn't say anything. Once my dad saw that I was crying, he started to as well. My mother quickly put a stop to any emotions by announcing that she had to have a milkshake. So we went across the street to McDonald's where my mom could drink her 'cancer milkshake.' "[3]

In the shadow of our cancer experience lurk some well-meaning bloopers coming in the form of comments, advice, religious and spiritual rhetoric, and just plain bonehead communication. It can be helpful to see how others have responded to uncomfortable conversations. You might find some useful lines that you can use in those instances when it's difficult to know what to say to a strange or thoughtless remark. And most important of all, sometimes you just need to laugh.

HOW WAS YOUR LIFE CHANGED AFTER CANCER? HOW WERE YOU CHANGED?

I asked a varied and small group of cancer survivors two questions: How was your life changed after cancer? And how were you changed? Here are some of their responses.

"For a while I was in the mode of 'take time to smell the roses,' but that went away and I think I went right back to being too busy."
—**Beth**

"It was during cancer treatment that I discovered qigong. Thinking it would keep me well and strong, I practiced it devoutly. When a cancer sister and fellow qigong practitioner had a recurrence and died, my qigong practice took a great blow. Looking back, I would say that I was operating on the belief that if I practiced

qigong, I would have a long, healthy life . . . be immortal. Suddenly I felt vulnerable, impermanent, mortal. Cancer, aging, it all reeks of impermanence."
—Diane

"I don't think much. There are moments that I realize that I should wake up and think: 'My life is a miracle.' I survived a cancer that kills most people. Yet, mostly I wake up and think: 'Where's the coffee?' I consider that a sign of a healthy attitude toward life and death."
—Julie

"I am still my charming, charismatic self."
—Len

DEALING WITH WHAT PEOPLE SAY

Some of the best things about what people say to people with cancer can be found online. The following statements come from Stupid Cancer (http://stupidcancer.org/), an Internet site for young people with cancer. They held an online contest, "Best Worst Cancer Lines" with a prize offer of a trip to Las Vegas for the winner. These lines came from some of the contestants.

"You don't look sick—you look so much better than I thought you would."

"I can relate—I'm having a horrible time getting rid of this flu."

"You're so lucky, you'll never have another period." (This said to a young woman who would never be able to conceive a child after a complete hysterectomy.)

I heard the following lines many times during my own experience with cancer. I suspect that you are familiar with them, too.

"I know just how you feel." (This statement usually precedes the person breaking into an hysterical crying jag while you stand by wondering if you should offer comfort or just run in the opposite direction as fast as you can.)

"You'll be fine." (This classic remark infuriated me every time I heard it. How the hell did anyone know that? In retrospect, it was probably related to my diagnosis of breast cancer, aka the *good* cancer.)

"Aren't you over this by now?" (This is often asked fairly soon after you've finished treatment.)

And this excerpt from *Mortality* by Christopher Hitchens is a personal favorite of mine. It describes an account of a conversation Hitchens had during a book signing event.

SHE: I was so sorry to hear you had been ill.

ME: Thank you for saying so.

SHE: A cousin of mine had cancer.

ME: Oh, I *am* sorry to hear that.

SHE: [*As the line of customers lengthens behind her*] Yes, in his liver.

ME: That's never good.

SHE: But it went away, after the doctors had told him it was incurable.

ME: Well, that's what we all want to hear.

SHE: [*With those further back in line now showing signs of impatience*] Yes. But then it came back much worse than before.

ME: Oh, how dreadful.

SHE: And then he died. It was agonizing. *Agonizing.* Seemed to take him forever.

ME: [*Beginning to search for words*] . . .

SHE: Of course, he was a lifelong homosexual.

ME: [*Not quite finding the words, and not wishing to sound stupid by echoing "of course"*] . . .

SHE: And his whole immediate family disowned him. He died virtually alone.

ME: Well, I hardly know what to . . .

SHE: Anyway, I just wanted you to know that I understand *exactly* what you are going through.[4]

WHAT PROVIDERS SAY

Healthcare providers can also be a source of frightening feedback. The following are some examples of interactions between patients and their providers.

"The next knucklehead I come in contact with is the radiation oncologist who asks me, while I am lying on the table being tattooed in preparation for my treatment, *what kind of radiation plan I would like.* He's the doctor, the expert, what are you asking me? I proceed to get off the table and call the angel doctor again. He tells me it is time to go to another oncologist."
—Pam L.

"I can remember one visit to the oncologist during or after my treatments, when I asked him (it was a him) what my chances would be if I discovered another lump in my other breast and he implied that it was probably all over for me."
—Beth

ADVICE

In general, people want to help. You may receive numerous suggestions and pieces of advice when you have cancer. Some of it is so farfetched that all you can do is nod and quietly laugh or groan inside yourself.

The following are anonymous advice comments quoted on various Internet sites:

"A friend of my sister's preschool teacher did an alternative treatment to chemotherapy, didn't lose her hair, and is just fine. Why don't you call her?"

"Don't wallow in your feelings."

"Being fat causes cancer, you should lose weight."

And finally, I offer Hitchens again with this fantastic example of advice giving:

"In Tumortown you sometimes feel you may expire from sheer *advice*. A lot of it comes free and unsolicited. I must, without delay, begin ingesting the granulated essence of the peach pit (or is the apricot?), a sovereign remedy known to ancient civilizations but now covered up by greedy modern doctors. Another correspondent urges heaping doses of testosterone supplements, perhaps as a morale-booster. Or I must find myself in an appropriately receptive mental state. Macrobiotic or vegan diets will be all I require for nourishment during this experience. . . . As against all that, I did get a kind note from a Cheyenne-Arapaho, a friend of mine, saying that everyone she knew who had resorted to tribal remedies had died almost immediately, and suggesting that if I was offered any Native American medicines I should 'move as fast as possible in the opposite direction.' Some advice can actually be taken."[5]

THE BUSINESS OF CANCER

Cancer has also become a big business, offering trinkets to those who are patients as well as their supporters. To be fair, these are often fundraising products designed to keep cancer programs running and fund research to help better understand and, hopefully, find a cure for cancer. Some people are upset by all the pink ribbons and paraphernalia, while others embrace pinkness in all its sparkly glory. Personally, I found that pink was not actually such a bad color for me (fashion sense being drilled into me at a very early age by my mother) and added more of it to my wardrobe. My friend, Diana, who died of melanoma, bemoaned the fact that her cancer color was black. I insisted that black was far more sophisticated than pink—"lucky her!"

P. J. O'Rourke shares his perspective on the colors of cancer in this quote: "I have, of all the inglorious things, a malignant hemorrhoid. What color bracelet does one wear for that? And where does one wear it? And what slogan is appropriate? Perhaps that slogan can be sewn in needlepoint around the ruffle on a cover for my embarrassing little donut buttocks pillow."[6]

Then there are the financial repercussions of illness in the United States, which is one of the leading causes of bankruptcy. Many of us continue to work, if we are able, to not put our families in a precarious financial position. For those who are unable to continue at their jobs, it can be a devastating financial experience that may take years to recover from. Many of the people I have spoken with have been severely affected by financial fallout. This is particularly true of underserved populations, again in the United States where healthcare is a for-profit business. The stress from money woes can be one of the most difficult aspects in survivorship. Once you are post-treatment, the bills start appearing regularly. In the years since I finished treatment for cancer, I have continued to have ongoing medical bills. At this point, they relate to the chronic damage from side effects of treatment as well as the continued follow-up tests, scans, and appointments that will be necessary for the rest of my life.

> "A hospital should also have a recovery room adjoining the cashier's office."
> **—Francis O'Walsh**[7]
>
> "I thought about how isolating it is to be sick in the US, everyone at work all the time, being home alone or driving to appointments alone in the middle of the day. Between appointments, meetings, clients, too many plates to keep in the air."
> **—Bonnie, friend**
>
> "I got the bill for my surgery. Now I know what those doctors were wearing masks for."
> **—James Boren**[8]

WHEN YOU DON'T RELATE TO RELIGION OR EMBRACE A SPIRITUAL PERSPECTIVE

Religious and spiritual beliefs are quite often related to healing from cancer as well as other illnesses. Memoirs and personal growth articles and books abound carrying strong religious messages. Prayer is highlighted in much of this literature, and we are often told to pray or that others are praying for us. Although I am not prone to jump on the organized religion bandwagon, I do believe that everyone has a right to their beliefs—as long as those beliefs don't become oppressive dogma that gets shoved down my throat. And I am appreciative of a prayer or any good thought on my behalf. Spiritually oriented groups are offered in many hospital and clinic settings, many of them based on a mindfulness model. All of this offers comfort except to those who really don't feel heard at all if they don't sing along with that tune. These folks are often labeled negative rather than accepted for their own lack of religious or spiritual beliefs. Although it has been shown that some type of spiritual outlook improves quality for those struggling with illness, this push to find redemption can actually be offensive to some people, and alternatives are important for those who prefer a more temporal view.

> "I sympathize afresh with the mighty Voltaire, who, when badgered on his deathbed and urged to renounce the devil, murmured that this was no time to be making enemies."
> **—Christopher Hitchens,** *Mortality*[9]

THE TYRANNY OF POSITIVE THINKING

The tyranny of positive thinking runs rampant in the cancer community. Although there is no conclusive evidence of stress, depression, or a specific personality type causing cancer, these dangerous judgments continue to exist and cause a great deal of personal pain to those struggling with illness. Self-blame and the idea that you somehow caused your cancer by not thinking the right way only clouds the truth that you did not choose this illness. Perhaps in that way, it is an antidote to helplessness or a modicum of certainty in an uncertain world. However, there are better ways to soothe the confusion of not knowing, of not having control, than dwelling on the unsolicited opinions of others, or even worse, beating yourself up with blame and shame.

Judgment and criticism are never found in the list of healing qualities nor is feeling bad about how well you are—or are not—holding up. In her book, *Strength Renewed: Meditations for Your Journey through Breast Cancer,* Shirley Corder writes, "Please don't preach at me—I feel bad enough already."[10]

Cancer seems to be a robust focus of the positive-thinking brigade. We don't seem to pressure people who have other equally life-threatening diseases to be positive. We don't tell them that their disease is a gift. Why is it that we insist on whitewashing cancer into some awesome life-changing window of opportunity?

"The failure to think positively can weigh on a cancer patient like a second disease," writes Barbara Ehrenreich in her book *Bright-Sided: How the Relentless Promotion of Positive Thinking Has Undermined America.*[11]

On the other side of the positive thinking coin is the tyranny of addressing cancer by being smart, sassy, and edgy. This import from the glib "get over it, don't wallow" school of thought creates guilt and shame for having lingering feelings, particularly in survivorship. The message is that something is pathologically wrong with you if you still feel worried, scared, sad, and the worst of all, depressed. You're supposed to be sexy and cool. Get a tattoo and go skydiving. The point seems to be that you need to impress others with your courage and moxie. It's become cool to act like it's all just a big joke.

Tell this to a stage IV colon cancer patient: "If I keep grinning maybe my inoperable colon cancer won't hurt so much."[12]

A cancer survivor recently said to me, "I thought I could go under it, I thought I could go around it, and then I realized that I had to go through it, and here I am."[13] The balance of dark and light, and the endeavor not only to stay alive but to make something out of a horrible experience, is an age-old tale of loss and redemption. Once you accept the challenge of the hero's journey, you will dive deep in stormy water, gasping for air, until you wash up on some new land that you didn't expect to arrive in. This is a deeply personal commitment, not a day trip to the beach.

The sooner we can acknowledge the underbelly of the cancer experience, the sooner we can balance the horror and the gift. Bitterness and overwhelming anxiety are merely plugged up emotions that haven't been allowed a scream or a howling cry. Yell, shout, cry, shiver—shake until you can't shake anymore. Then rest, and move on. Understand that all those stupid comments people make come from not knowing what to say. I've come to realize that the remark which annoyed me the most, "you'll be fine," was only the well-meaning and frightened wish of those around me that I would be fine. And my heartfelt response to them is, "Thank you for believing that I will be fine. Now leave me alone."

> *Here's a fact: Some people want to live more*
> *Than others do. Some can withstand any horror.*
> *While others will easily surrender*
> *To thirst, hunger, and extremes of weather.*
> *In Utah, one man carried another*

Man on his back like a conjoined brother
And crossed twenty-five miles of desert
To safety. Can you imagine the hurt?
Do you think you could be that good and strong?
Yes, yes, *you think, but you're probably wrong.*
—Sherman Alexie, "Survivorman"[14]

"I have Chemo Bran . . . Brian . . . Brain . . ."
—seen on a T-shirt

WORKBOOK SECTION: A PLACE FOR YOU TO SHOUT AND SCREAM OUT LOUD!

You can use this space to vent your thoughts and feelings without censoring or softening your comments. Some questions that might help you get started:

- What's the dumbest thing anyone has ever said to you?
- What remarks or questions made you feel angry?
- What remarks or questions really hurt your feelings?
- What's the funniest line that someone has said to you?
- Talk about the times when really horrible predicaments become something to laugh about.

Give yourself permission to let loose!

NOTES

1. Ellen Bass, "French Chocolates" in *Like a Beggar* (Port Townsend, WA: Copper Canyon Press, 2014), 20. Used by permission of The Permissions Company, Inc., on behalf of Copper Canyon Press, www.coppercanyonpress.org. © 2014 by Ellen Bass.

2. John Green, *The Fault in Our Stars* (New York: Penguin, 2012), 217.

3. Personal interview with the author.

4. Christopher Hitchens, *Mortality* (New York: Twelve, 2012), 38–39. Used by permission of Twelve, an imprint of Grand Central Publishing. All rights reserved. © 2012 by Christopher Hitchens.

5. Hitchens, *Mortality*, 28–29.

6. P. J. O'Rourke, "Give Me Liberty and Give Me Death," *Los Angeles Times*, September 28, 2008, www.latimes.com/la-oe-orourke28-2008sep28-story.html. Used by permission of P. J. O'Rourke. Agreement facilitated by agent Bob Dattila and Greater Talent Network.

7. Francis O'Walsh, izQuotes.com, http://izquotes.com/quote/297490, accessed October 5, 2016.

8. James H. Boren, BrainyQuote.com, Xplore Inc, 2016, www.brainyquote.com/quotes/quotes/j/jameshbor106706.html, accessed October 5, 2016.

9. Hitchens, *Mortality*, 17.

10. Shirley Corder, *Strength Renewed: Meditations for Your Journey through Breast Cancer* (Grand Rapids, MI: Revell, 2012), 206.

11. Barbara Ehrenreich, *Bright-Sided: How the Relentless Promotion of Positive Thinking Has Undermined America* (New York: Metropolitan, 2009), 43. Used by permission of ICM. All rights reserved.

12. Tony Millionaire, *Maakies* (Seattle, WA: Fantagraphic Books, 2000). Used by permission of Tony Millionaire.

13. Personal interview with the author.

14. Sherman Alexie, "Survivorman," *New Yorker*, June 8, 2009, www.newyorker.com/magazine/2009/06/08/survivorman. Used by permission of the author. © 2009 by Sherman Alexie.

EPILOGUE

ENDINGS AND BEGINNINGS

WHAT WOULD YOU DO IF YOU KNEW you had only one more day, one last week, or one month to live? There's a philosophy that suggests that if you live each day as if it were your last, you become more alive, take more risks, and discover what you really want to do with whatever time you're given. You may shed your accepted and familiar skin in favor of becoming who you have always wanted to be, who you truly are. Workshops often pose the theoretical question, "What would you do if you only had a year to live?" People pay money to spend a weekend *imagining* that they are dying so that they may reflect on what they might do differently, what choices they would make, what dreams they might want to make come true. Some of us didn't take this course as an elective.

You didn't sign up for the course, but for the rest of your life, you'll be in this class. You have reached the end of this book, but it's not the end of your story. Yours is a story that began without you knowing where it would take you. As the tale continues to be told, there will be milestones and anniversaries, celebrations and disappointments, and sometimes just a feeling of overwhelming and welcome relief that you're still around. When you approach these touchstones and arrive at various checkpoints, thoughts and feelings may arise. The following are some examples of key times that can be evocative.

- Medical follow-up appointments can trigger anxiety and memories of past experiences.
- Diagnostic tests and scans can arouse fears and feelings.
- Blood draws can spark concerns.
- Aches, pains, fatigue, and odd unexplainable symptoms can throw you into doubt, dread, and confusion.
- The diagnosis of another person can bring up fears of recurrence of your cancer.

Exams will remind you of those first tests, the scan that showed something that shouldn't have been there, the phone call you'll never forget. Old demons will rear their heads in your dreams, make for sweaty palms and scary doubts, and the wait for results will always seem endless.

You can find both solace and insight in these moments by returning to the story templates and continuing your process of survivorship. These are the junctures when you may revisit your workbooks, continue your exploration, and create your story anew. You can refer back to this resource for support when important milestones occur.

- The anniversary of your diagnosis
- The date you started treatment
- The day you finished treatment
- A decrease in your medical appointments
- The diagnosis or death of another person from cancer

Benchmarks such as the anniversary of a diagnosis, remembering when you started treatment, or marking the date you finished treatment can be a time for you to contemplate where you are now, as well as an opportunity to reflect on where you have been. It can be disconcerting when you are released from care by your doctor; you can turn to these templates as a way to find your own structure. You can use the questions provided by the templates to help you modify your goals and revise your intentions. You may return to this resource as something to grab onto when you need comfort or have to face a challenge.

If you have been helped, you may find yourself passing the book to a friend, a family member, or someone you meet in the waiting room. This can be something to continue to share with yourself as well as with others. Because from the moment you started this book and began finding a way to voice your story, your life has changed. You have changed. The story that you told and the story that you tell today will not be the same as the one you will tell a year from now. Hopefully, there will be many more chapters in your life. Even now, in this moment, you are choosing and creating the story of your life.

As of this writing, it's been close to nine years since I finished treatment for cancer. I'm having a pretty good run. I've seen my son graduate from middle school, high school, and if all goes according to plan (a plan not just related to me and any kind of cancer but to the plans of a twenty-three-year-old male), from college this year. I've had adventures both at home and in my travels. I've celebrated twenty-five years of marriage and sixty-five years on the planet. As a psychotherapist, I am now known as someone who specializes in working with cancer patients and their communities. I call this "the specialty that chose me" and, believe me, I did not plan on this one! I have met and worked with courageous cancer patients and their families and collaborated with amazing providers, all of whom have taught me profound lessons and given me far more than I have offered them. I have been privileged to attend to the needs of underserved communities whose struggles must be understood and honored.

I've learned that not everything makes sense and that *even* I cannot change that.

I no longer worry about what people think of me. Another point that *even* I cannot control.

I now believe that "what the hell" usually is the way to go.

Alan Watts said, "The only way to make sense out of change is to plunge into it, move with it, and join the dance."[1] I don't know why I became one of the statistics that no one wants to be. I don't know if cancer will come back and grab me, or if one day I'll simply nod off with a dribble of Cream of Wheat running down my wrinkled, ancient chin. What I do know is that I am grateful to be given the chance to change and to stick around plunging into the next unknown moment. I'm glad I still get to join in the dance—even though it's not always pretty or sexy. I've had to dance for my life, and so have you. I know that I'll keep on dancing and speaking my story for the rest of my days, and I wish the same for you.

NOTE

1. Alan W. Watts, *The Wisdom of Insecurity: A Message for an Age of Anxiety*, 2nd ed. (New York: Vintage, 2011), 43.

RESOURCES

I would recommend that you check out your local resources as they will usually be able to provide you with more personal care and attention than some of the larger, national organizations. You can find them by asking your providers for referrals as well as by searching online. For example, search "cancer survivor support" followed by typing in the area where you live (e.g., "cancer survivor support San Francisco Bay Area"). By looking locally, you can connect with others in your area.

I also recommend online resources as a wonderful way to connect. I was the last person who would have expected to find such a satisfying community online, but those I have met online have proved to be companions and helpmates on the path. Search by looking at resources by type of cancer, age group, and events that interest you. You may be surprised to find a plethora of creative outlets to choose from. I include some of the "heavy hitters" for cancer resources that I find useful. Beware of sites that promise too much or frighten you with generalized statistics—be a smart consumer of both online and in-person resources—check them out carefully.

- Cancer Survivors Network—American Cancer Society
  http://csn.cancer.org
- National Cancer Institute (NCI)
  www.cancer.gov/about-cancer/coping/survivorship
- Cancer Support Community
  www.cancersupportcommunity.org
- National Coalition for Cancer Survivorship (NCCS)
  www.canceradvocacy.org
- American Psychosocial Oncology Society (APOS)
  https://apos-society.org
- International Psychosocial Oncology Society (IPOS)
  www.ipos-society.org/for-patients/resources-for-patients-and-families
- Cancer.Net
  www.cancer.net
- National Cancer Survivorship Resource Center
  www.cancer.org/treatment/survivorshipduringandaftertreatment/
  nationalcancersurvivorshipresourcecenter/index
- LIVESTRONG
  www.livestrong.org
- Casting for Recovery: "The mission of Casting for Recovery (CfR) is to enhance the quality of life of women with breast cancer through a unique program that combines breast cancer education and peer support with the therapeutic sport of fly fishing. The retreats offer opportunities for women to find inspiration, discover renewed energy for life, and experience healing connections with other women and nature. CfR's retreats are open to breast cancer survivors of all ages, in all stages of treatment and recovery, and are free to participants."
  https://castingforrecovery.org
- Reel Recovery: "Reel Recovery was founded in 2003 by a group of avid fly-fishers, inspired by their fishing buddy's ongoing battle with brain cancer. Witnessing firsthand the beneficial impact fly-fishing provided their friend, they created Reel Recovery to provide the same opportunity for other men battling the disease. Combining expert fly-fishing instruction with directed 'courageous conversations,' the organization provides men with all forms of cancer a unique opportunity to share their stories, learn a new skill, form lasting friendships and gain renewed hope as they confront the challenges of cancer."
  http://reelrecovery.org
- Commonweal Cancer Help Program: "The Commonweal Cancer Help Program (CCHP) is a week-long retreat for people with cancer. Our goal is to help participants live better and, where possible, longer lives. CCHP addresses the unmet needs of people with cancer. These include finding balanced information on choices in healing, mainstream and complementary therapies; exploring emotional and spiritual dimensions of cancer;

discovering that illness can sometimes lead to a richer and fuller life; and experiencing genuine community with others facing a cancer diagnosis."
www.commonweal.org/program/cchp

- StupidCancer: "Stupid Cancer proudly supports a global network of patients, survivors, caregivers, providers and advocates to ensure that no one affected by young adult cancer go unaware of the age-appropriate resources they are entitled to so they can get busy living. Our innovative and multi-award-winning programs—such as CancerCon, Instapeer, The OMG! Cancer Summit for Young Adults, The Stupid Cancer Road Trip, The Stupid Cancer Store and many others—have brought the cause of 'cancer under 40' to the national spotlight and rallied a brand new generation of activists to give a much needed voice to our forgotten population."
http://stupidcancer.org

RESOURCES FOR WORKING WITH TRAUMA

All of the following organizations have practitioners in different areas of both the United States and throughout the rest of the world. Psychotherapists who are comfortable and familiar with issues of illness and survivorship can be of service to you as well as to your family. You can also ask your physician for a referral. Take your time to find the right connection with the practitioner you choose.

- Somatic Experiencing is a method developed by Peter Levine, PhD. There are certified practitioners of this method in many areas of the world.
www.traumahealing.com
- The Sensorimotor Psychotherapy Institute is run by Pat Ogden, PhD. This type of therapy "provides a bridge between traditional psychotherapy and body-oriented therapies."
www.sensorimotorpsychotherapy.org
- The Hakomi Institute is also an excellent option for those looking to work with their trauma through the body–mind connection.
www.hakomiinstitute.com
- The Trauma Center at Justice Resource Institute was founded by Dr. Bessel van der Kolk, "an internationally recognized leader in the field of psychological trauma."
www.traumacenter.org
- Yoga4Cancer was founded by Tari Prinster, who is a cancer survivor, yoga teacher, and author.
http://y4c.com
- The Integrative Restoration Institute (IRI) is under the direction of Richard Miller, PhD. IRI helps "people resolve their pain and suffering by *rediscovering their essential wholeness*. . .trauma and difficult life situations are then met with a deeply wise and compassionate response."
www.irest.us
- The United States Association for Body Psychotherapy offers a comprehensive online practitioner directory.
www.usabp.org

RECOMMENDED READING

Abel, Emily K., and Saskia K. Subramanian. *After the Cure: The Untold Stories of Breast Cancer Survivors.* New York: New York University Press, 2008.

Chödrön, Pema. *Living Beautifully with Uncertainty and Change.* Boston: Shambhala, 2012.

de Hennezel, Marie. *Intimate Death: How the Dying Teach Us How to Live.* New York: Vintage, 1998.

Eggers, Dave. *A Heartbreaking Work of Staggering Genius.* New York: Vintage, 2001.

Gonzales, Laurence. *Surviving Survival: The Art and Science of Resilience.* New York: W. W. Norton, 2013.

Kornfield, Jack. *A Path with Heart: A Guide through the Perils and Promises of Spiritual Life.* New York: Bantam, 1993.

Levine, Peter. *Waking the Tiger: Healing Trauma.* Berkeley, CA: North Atlantic Books, 1997.

Pogrebin, Letty Cotton. *How to Be a Friend to a Friend Who's Sick.* Philadelphia: Perseus, 2014.

Watts, Alan W. *The Wisdom of Insecurity: A Message for an Age of Anxiety.* New York: Vintage, 2011.

BIBLIOGRAPHY

Alexie, Sherman. "Survivorman." *New Yorker* (June 8, 2009). www.newyorker.com/magazine/2009/06/08/survivorman.

American Cancer Society. *Living with Uncertainty: The Fear of Cancer Recurrence*. Last revised June 19, 2013. www.cancer.org/acs/groups/cid/documents/webcontent/002014-pdf.pdf.

American Psychiatric Association. *Diagnostic and Statistical Manual of Mental Disorders*. 5th ed. Arlington, VA: American Psychiatric Association, 2013.

American Society of Clinical Oncology. "Post-Traumatic Stress Disorder and Cancer." Cancer.net (January 2016). www.cancer.net/survivorship/life-after-cancer/post-traumatic-stress-disorder-and-cancer.

Atwood, Margaret. "A Boat." In *Selected Poems II: Poems Selected and New, 1976–1986*, p. 120. Boston: Houghton Mifflin, 1987.

Bass, Ellen. "French Chocolates." In *Like a Beggar*, 20. Port Townsend, WA: Copper Canyon Press, 2014.

Berra, Yogi. *The Yogi Book*. New York: Workman, 2010.

Bly, Robert. "The Blind Old Man." In *Talking into the Ear of a Donkey*, 29. New York: W. W. Norton, 2011.

Bugental, James F. T. *The Art of the Psychotherapist: How to Develop the Skills That Take Psychotherapy beyond Science*. New York: W. W. Norton, 1987.

Bugental, James F. T. *Psychotherapy and Process: The Fundamentals of an Existential-Humanistic Approach*. 3rd ed. New York: McGraw-Hill, 1978.

Bugental, James F. T. *The Search for Authenticity: An Existential-Analytical Approach to Psychotherapy*. Manchester, NH: Irvington, 1981.

Burroughs, William S. *Junky*. New York: Grove Press, 2003.

Chödrön, Pema. *When Things Fall Apart: Heart Advice for Difficult Times*. Boulder, CO: Shambhala, 1997.

Collins, Billy. "My Number." In *The Apple That Astonished Paris*, 54. Fayetteville, AR: University of Arkansas Press, 1996.

Corder, Shirley. *Strength Renewed: Meditations for Your Journey through Breast Cancer*. Grand Rapids, MI: Revell, 2012.

Cornwall, Deborah J. "How Cancer Caregivers Heal." Cancer Knowledge Network (August 1, 2013). https://cancerkn.com/how-cancer-caregivers-heal/.

Ehrenreich, Barbara. *Bright-Sided: How the Relentless Promotion of Positive Thinking Has Undermined America*. New York: Metropolitan, 2009.

50/50. Directed by Jonathan Levine. Santa Monica, CA: Summit Entertainment, 2011.

Gibran, Kahlil. "On Death." In *The Prophet*, 80. New York: Knopf, 1973.

Green, John. *The Fault in Our Stars*. New York: Penguin, 2012.

Handler, Evan. *It's Only Temporary: The Good News and Bad News about Being Alive*. New York: Riverhead Books, 2008.

Hitchens, Christopher. *Mortality*. New York: Twelve, 2012.

Jay, Jeffrey. "Terrible Knowledge." *Family Therapy Networker* (November/December 1991): 21.

Joseph, Stephen. *What Doesn't Kill Us: The New Psychology of Posttraumatic Growth*. New York: Basic Books, 2011.

Kooser, Ted. "At the Cancer Clinic." In *Delights & Shadows*, 7. Port Townsend, WA: Copper Canyon Press, 2004.

Kornfield, Jack. *Buddha's Little Instruction Book*. New York: Bantam, 1994.

Kunitz, Stanley. "The Layers." In *The Collected Poems*, 217–18. New York: W. W. Norton, 2000.

Lederberg, Marguerite S., and Jimmie C. Holland. "Supportive Psychotherapy in Cancer Care: An Essential Ingredient of All Therapy." In *Handbook of Psychotherapy in Cancer Care*, edited by Maggie Watson and David W. Kissane, 1–14. Chichester, UK: Wiley-Blackwell, 2011.

Lent, Robert W. "Restoring Emotional Well-Being: A Theoretical Model." In *Handbook of Cancer Survivorship*, edited by Michael Feuerstein, 231–47. New York: Springer, 2007.

LeShan, Lawrence. *Cancer as a Turning Point: A Handbook for People with Cancer, Their Families, and Health Professionals*. 2nd rev. ed. New York: Plume, 1994.

LeShan, Lawrence. *You Can Fight for Your Life: Emotional Factors in the Treatment of Cancer.* Guilford, CT: M. Evans, 1980.

Levertov, Denise. "Sojourns in the Parallel World." In *Sands of the Well*, 49. New York: New Directions, 1998.

Levine, Ondrea. *The Healing I Took Birth For: Practicing the Art of Compassion.* rev. ed. Newburyport, MA: Weiser Books, 2015.

Levine, Peter A. *In an Unspoken Voice: How the Body Releases Trauma and Restores Goodness.* Berkeley, CA: North Atlantic Books, 2010.

LiveStrong Foundation. *Fear of Recurrence.* 2011. www.fredhutch.org/content/dam/public/Treatment-Suport/survivorship/Healthy-Links/Fear%20of%20Recurrence.pdf.

May, Rollo. *Freedom and Destiny.* New York: W. W. Norton, 1981.

Miller, Kenneth, Brian Merry, and Joan Miller. "Seasons of Survivorship Revisited." *Cancer Journal* 14, no. 6 (November/December, 2008): 369–74. doi:10.1097/PPO.0b013e31818edf60.

Millionaire, Tony. *Maakies.* Seattle, WA: Fantagraphic Books, 2000.

Mullan, Fitzhugh. "Seasons of Survival: Reflections of a Physician with Cancer." *New England Journal of Medicine* 313, no. 4 (July 25, 1985): 270–73. doi:10.1056/NEJM198507253130421.

National Cancer Institute. *Facing Forward: Life after Cancer Treatment.* rev. ed. National Institutes of Health Publication no. 14-2424. Washington, DC: U.S. Department of Health and Human Services, 2014.

O'Donohue, John. "The Question Holds the Lantern." Accessed September 27, 2016. www.john-odonohue.com/words/question.

Oliver, Mary. "The Uses of Sorrow." In *Thirst*, 52. Boston: Beacon Press, 2006.

PDQ Supportive and Palliative Care Editorial Board. "PDQ Cancer-Related Post-traumatic Stress." (Bethesda, MD: National Cancer Institute). Updated January 7, 2015. www.cancer.gov/about-cancer/coping/survivorship/new-normal/ptsd-hp-pdq.

Peabody, Francis W. "The Care of the Patient." *The Journal of the American Medical Association* 88, no. 12 (March 19, 1927): 877–82. doi:10.1001/jama.1927.02680380001001.

Plumly, Stanley. "Cancer." In *Orphan Hours*, 26–27. New York: W. W. Norton, 2012.

Quality of Life Research Unit. "Quality of Life Model." University of Toronto, Ontario. Accessed September 29, 2016. http://sites.utoronto.ca/qol/qol_model.htm.

Radner, Gilda. *It's Always Something.* New York: Simon & Schuster, 1989.

Rakoff, David. *Half Empty.* New York: Doubleday, 2010.

Rogers, Fred. *Life's Journeys According to Mr. Rogers: Things to Remember along the Way.* New York: Hyperion Books, 2005.

Seuss, Dr. *Horton Hears a Who!* New York: Random House, 1954.

Siegel, Bernie. *Love, Medicine & Miracles: Lessons Learned about Self-Healing from a Surgeon's Experience with Exceptional Patients.* New York: HarperPerennial, 1990.

Stafford, William. "Any Time." In *The Way It Is: New & Selected Poems*, 127. Minneapolis, MN: Graywolf Press, 1998.

Stafford, William. "In the White Sky." In *Stories That Could Be True: New and Collected Poems*, 217. New York: Harper & Row, 1973.

Stanton, Annette L. "What Happens Now? Psychosocial Care for Cancer Survivors after Medical Treatment Completion." *Journal of Clinical Oncology* 30, no. 11 (2012): 1215–20. doi:10.1200/JCO.2011.39.7406.

Tedeschi, Richard G., and Lawrence G. Calhoun. "The Foundations of Posttraumatic Growth: New Considerations." *Psychological Inquiry* 15, no. 1 (2004): 93.

Tedeschi, Richard G., and Lawrence G. Calhoun. *Trauma and Transformation: Growing in the Aftermath of Suffering.* Thousand Oaks, CA: Sage, 1995.

Wallace, Ronald. "The Truth." In *Long for This World: New and Selected Poems*, 98. Pittsburgh, PA: University of Pittsburg Press, 2003.

"Warfield Theobald Longcope." In *The Oxford Dictionary of Medical Quotations*, edited by Peter McDonald, 61. Oxford, UK: Oxford University Press, 2004.

Watts, Alan W. *The Wisdom of Insecurity: A Message for an Age of Anxiety.* 2nd ed. New York: Vintage, 2011.

Weaver, Ryan Rose. "What Should Siblings Do in the Face of Cancer?" Roswell Park Cancer Institute (blog). Accessed October 6, 2016. www.roswellpark.org/cancertalk/201302/what-should-siblings-do-face-cancer.

Yalom, Irvin. D. *Staring at the Sun: Overcoming the Terror of Death*. San Francisco: Jossey-Bass, 2009.

Zak, Paul J. "How Stories Change the Brain." *Greater Good: The Science of a Meaningful Life* (December 17, 2013). http://greatergood.berkeley.edu/article/item/how_stories_change_brain.

ABOUT THE AUTHOR

Cheryl Krauter, MFT, is an existential humanistic psychotherapist with more than thirty-five years of experience in the field of depth psychology and human consciousness. She integrates her experience as a depth psychotherapist with her personal journey as a cancer survivor. Krauter began working with people in various stages of a cancer diagnosis after her own experience and has presented numerous talks and workshops on living with the uncertainty of life-threatening illness. She advocates for humanizing cancer care by attending to the need for the emotional healing of a cancer diagnosis. www.cherylkrauter.com www.cancersurvivorsupport.com

INDEX